Health

Made Simple!

by Christine Lauren

First Edition Published April 2017
independently through Createspace.com
Charleston, South Carolina

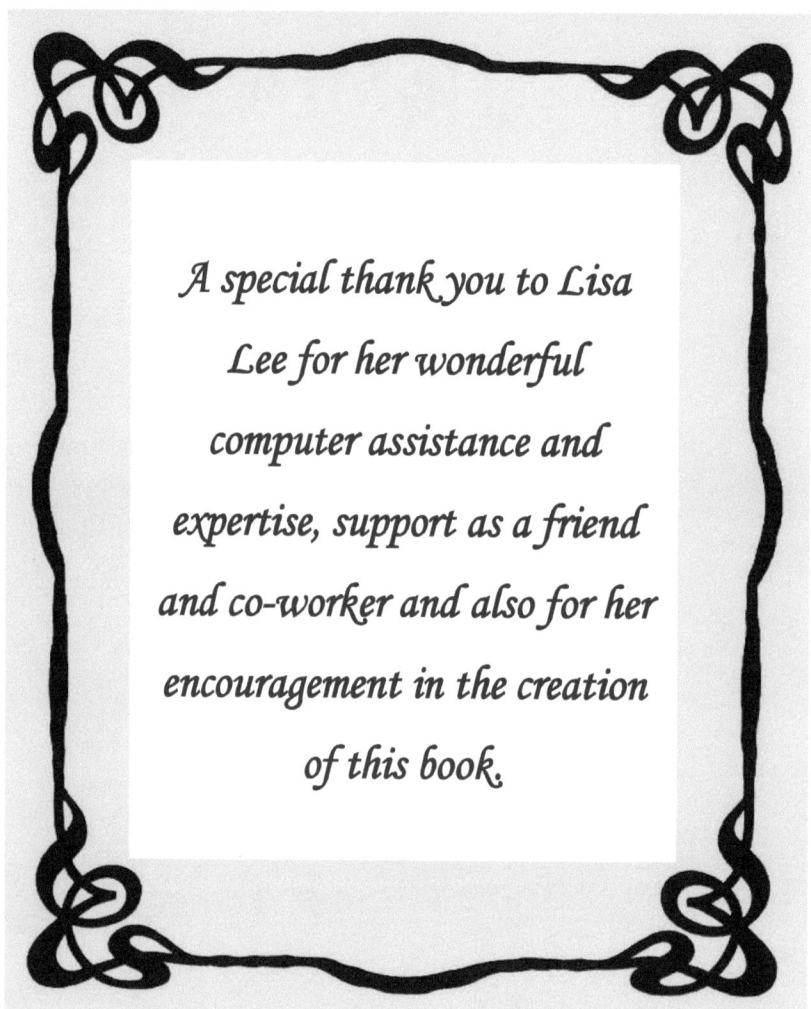

A special thank you to Lisa Lee for her wonderful computer assistance and expertise, support as a friend and co-worker and also for her encouragement in the creation of this book.

Disclaimer: This book is written for educational purposes only.
It is not intended to diagnose or prescribe in regard to any specific malady. It is up to the discretion of the reader to apply any or all of the information provided and to consult his or her attending physician regarding any interaction with drugs or treatment already being taken.

To order, search by author's name and title at www.amazon.com and or use this web address www.createspace.com/6112786 as an URL. Do not put in the search bar.

Contact author at feetadancing@gmail.com

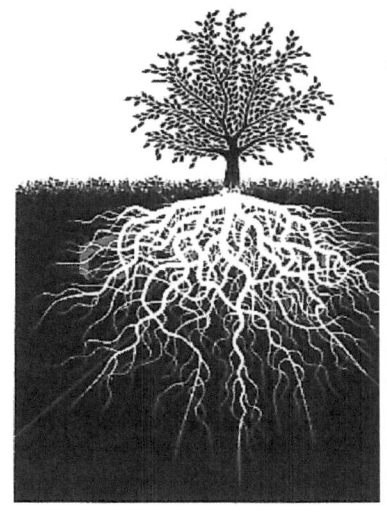

You may be asking, "How does a tree with a profound root system relate to my health?"

In Jeremiah 17:7-8 it says, "Blessed is the man that trusts in the Lord and whose hope the Lord is. For he shall be as a tree planted by the water that spreads out her roots by the river..."

I believe the Bible is the Word of God and that it is alive and powerful. For that reason, I reference it in this book because it is my foundation.

A healthy tree is well watered deep below the surface of the earth at its very roots. A healthy body needs to be well hydrated at its deepest cellular level as well.

A healthy tree grows in good soil that is rich in minerals. A healthy body needs to be fed good, living food to be nourished and sustained. A healthy body also needs minerals that energize the bloodstream because as declared in the Bible, the life is in the blood.

To remain healthy, a tree needs to be cared for. If a worm is eating its leaves, or a parasitic blight is eroding its vast root system, then those predators need to be brought to a halt. In the human body, when there are pollutants or parasites that are warring against its natural, healthy state, then those predators need to be exterminated as well.

The premise of having only four basic steps to great health comes from the simplicity of truth found in the Word of God.

It would be endless if we looked only at symptoms of the tree being sick. But if we look at the quality of the water source, the richness of the soil and the minerals in the soil and then do what ever we need to do to counteract the attack of damaging parasites or pollution, then it becomes a **simple four-step process**.

So it is with the human body. If we focus on symptoms, the battle is baffling and never ending. If we correct or enhance the basics, then a sturdy and enduring foundation for good health is laid.

The four steps I am sharing with you build that foundation: **Quality water, a potentially life-changing super food, a stunning mineral source and a profoundly effective solution to eliminating pathogens from the body.** This strong foundation is time-tested and based on what is true for the human body. I can make that statement because I have personally lived this process. When I was twenty and working in a health food store, the Lord let me know that if I did not become a heath nut, I would either die or be in a wheel chair. That was fifty years ago. For that reason, I am sharing with you what has most fundamentally enabled me to be strong and healthy over all these years. These four steps have given me a four-note song that has a happy tune.

Best wishes as you gain health made simple!

Christine Lauren
April, 2017

FOUR STEPS TO GOOD HEALTH

STEP ONE: QUALITY WATER

STEP TWO: GREEN SUPER FOOD

STEP THREE: HIMALAYAN SALT

STEP FOUR: PATHOGEN ELIMINATION

Water is so important that without it we would not exist.

We are about 70 % water. *Babies are 80% water. The elderly are 50% water. The brain is 90% water!* **It has been found that people in care facilities exhibiting signs of Alzheimer's disease often regain their mental faculties when they drink enough water.**

What Does Water do for You?

Forms saliva (digestion)

Keeps mucousal membranes moist

Allows body's cells to grow, reproduce and survive

Flushes body waste, mainly in urine

Lubricates joints

Water is the major component of most body parts

Needed by the brain to manufacture hormones and neurotransmitters

Regulates body temperature (sweating and respiration)

Acts as a shock absorber for brain and spinal cord

Converts food to components needed for survival - digestion

Helps deliver oxygen all over the body

My routine: I drink two 16-ounce glasses of water upon rising. Then I wait 45 minutes before brushing my teeth or eating anything. I put 1 teaspoon of Himalayan salt in the second glass. Salt is the third component to good health talked more about later. The Japanese Medical Society bases this regime on studies. Flushing the body in the morning purifies the body and makes *the colon more effective in forming fresh new blood.* The Bible says "the life is in the blood" in Leviticus 17:11. *I have not been sick once since faithfully following this routine!*

Things to know about body chemistry:

Our bodies are fearfully and wonderfully made, designed to have optimum heath at a pH of 6.5 to 7.5. pH is "potential hydrogen" or the ability to attract hydrogen.

At a pH of 7.5 (alkaline) *cancer cells, which are acidic, die.* **At a pH of 5.8 (acidic) cancer cells begin to form.** At a pH of 3.5 (acidic) the human body cannot sustain life. Diet colas have a pH of 3.3 rivaling the pH of battery acid at 1.0. *The body will put everything else at risk to maintain the pH of the blood at 7.365.*

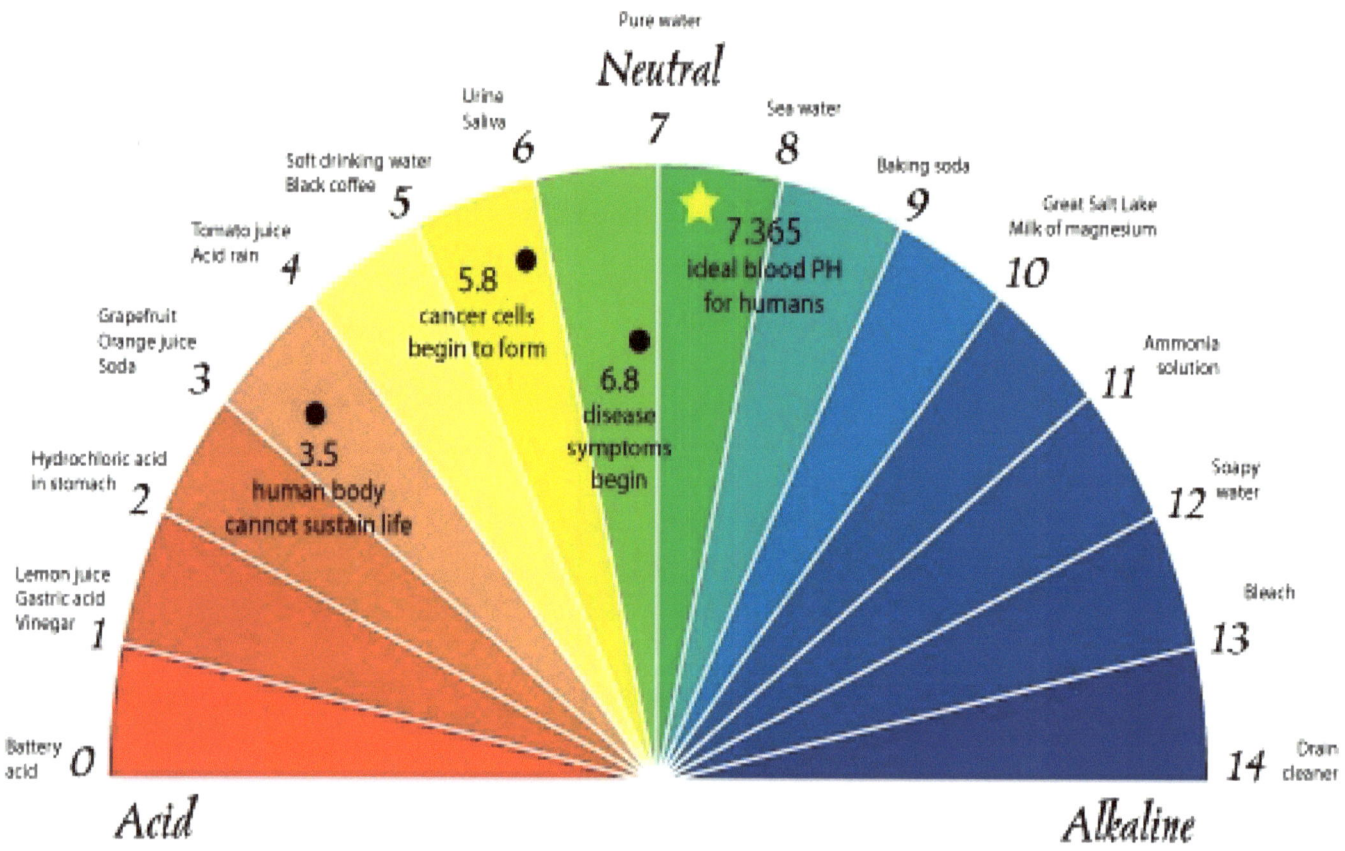

Note: According to www.angelfire.com,

"When the pH of a cancer cell goes above 7.5 it dies and if it goes above 8.0 it will die in a matter of hours."

It also states,
"Cancer cells live in an acidic environment,
but perish in an alkaline, high pH, environment."

pH Food Chart

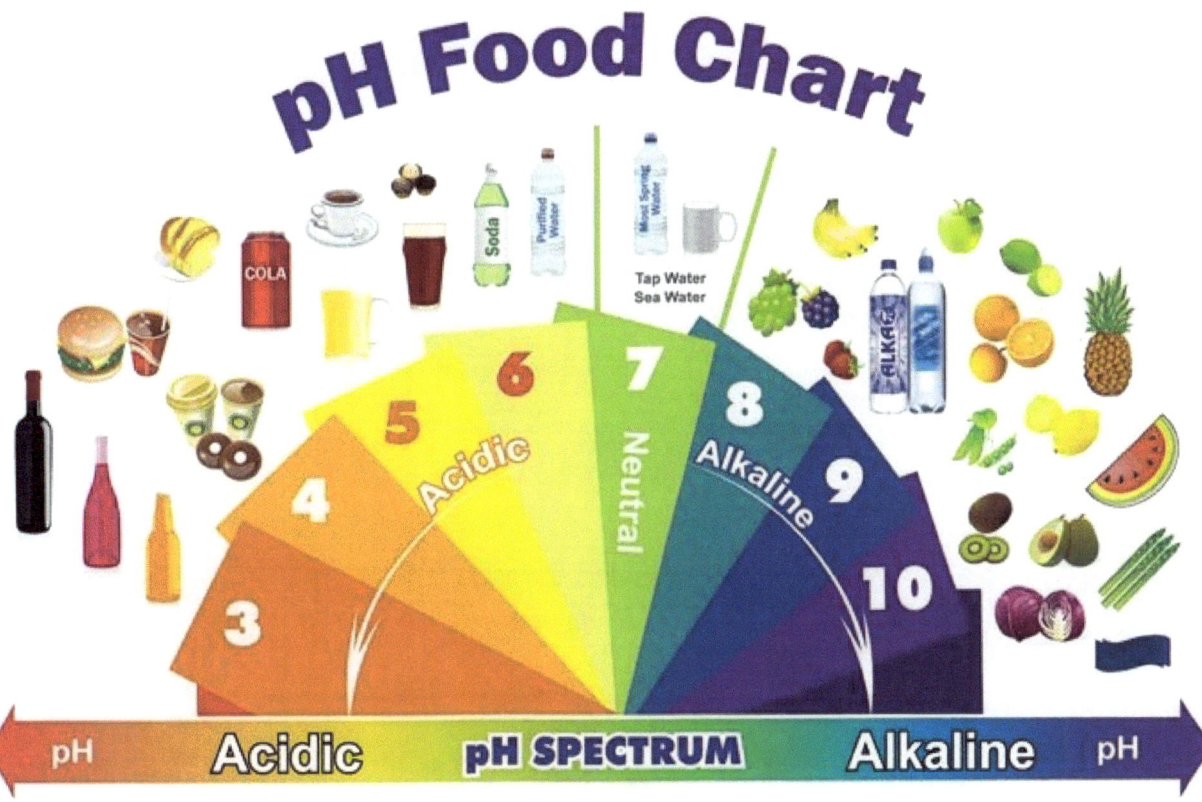

Acidic   **pH SPECTRUM**   **Alkaline**

3 — Carbonated Water, Club Soda, Energy Drinks

4 — Popcorn, Cream Cheese, Buttermilk, Prunes Pastries, Pasta, Cheese, Pork, Beer, Wine, Black Tea, Pickles, Chocolate, Roasted Nuts, Vinegar, Sweet and Low, Equal, Nutra Sweet

5 — Most Purified Water, Distilled Water, Coffee, Sweetened Fruit Juice, Pistachios, Beef, White Bread, Peanuts, Nuts, Wheat, Blueberries, Cranberries

6 — Fruit Juices, Most Grains, Eggs, Fish, Tea, Cooked Beans, Cooked Spinach, Soy Milk, Coconut, Lima Beans, Plums, Brown Rice, Barley, Cocoa, Oats, Liver, Oyster, Salmon

Neutral pH

7 — Most Tap Water, Most Spring Water, Sea Water, River Water

8 — Apples, Almonds, Avocados, Tomatoes, Grapefruit, Corn, Mushrooms, Turnip, Olive, Soybeans, Peaches, Bell Pepper, Radish, Pineapple, Cherries, Wild Rice, Apricot, Strawberries, Bananas

9 — Avocados, Green Tea, Lettuce, Celery, Peas, Sweet Potatoes, Egg Plant, Green Beans, Beets, Blueberries, Pears, Grapes, Kiwi, Melons, Tangerines, Figs, Dates, Mangoes, Papayas

10 — Spinach, Broccoli, Artichoke, Brussel Sprouts, Cabbage, Cauliflower, Carrots, Cucumbers, Lemons, Limes, Seaweed, Asparagus, Radish, Kale, Collard Greens, Onion

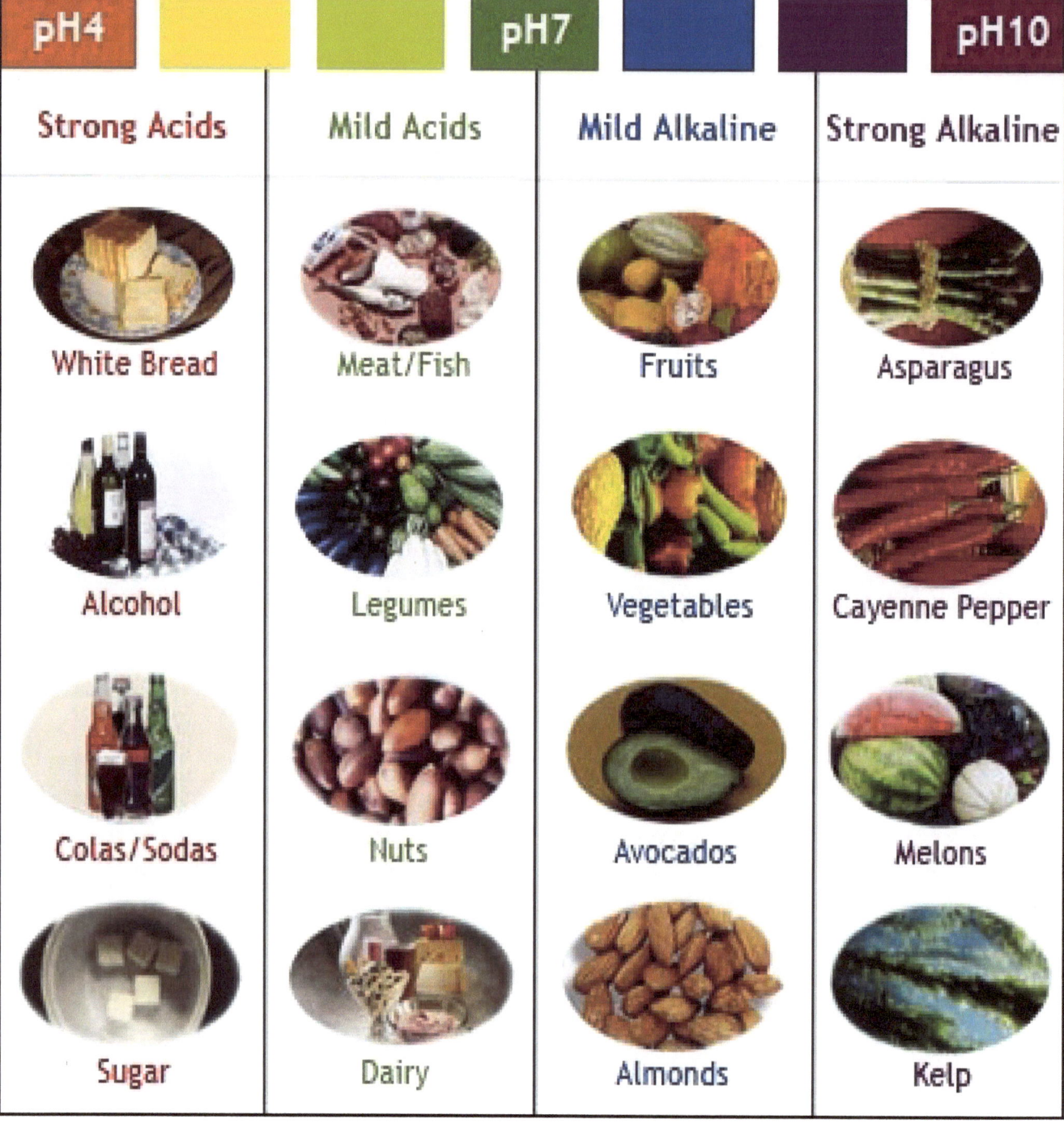

pH4			pH7			pH10
Strong Acids		**Mild Acids**		**Mild Alkaline**		**Strong Alkaline**
White Bread		Meat/Fish		Fruits		Asparagus
Alcohol		Legumes		Vegetables		Cayenne Pepper
Colas/Sodas		Nuts		Avocados		Melons
Sugar		Dairy		Almonds		Kelp

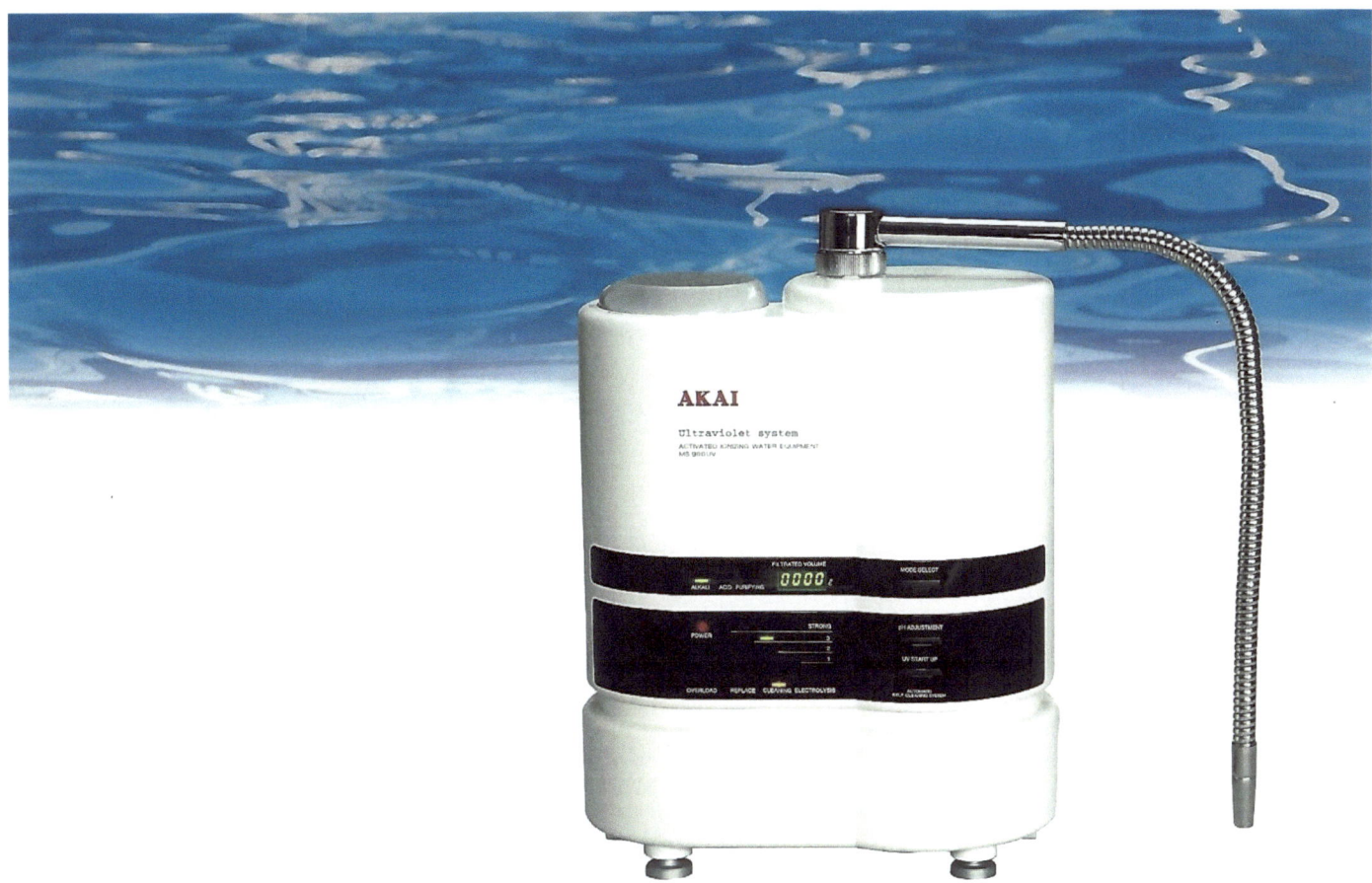

IONIZER PLUS®
WATER ELECTROLYZER

YOUR SOLUTION FOR WHOLE BODY HEALTH

Reverse the conditions that inhibit the body's own mechanisms for maintaining good health

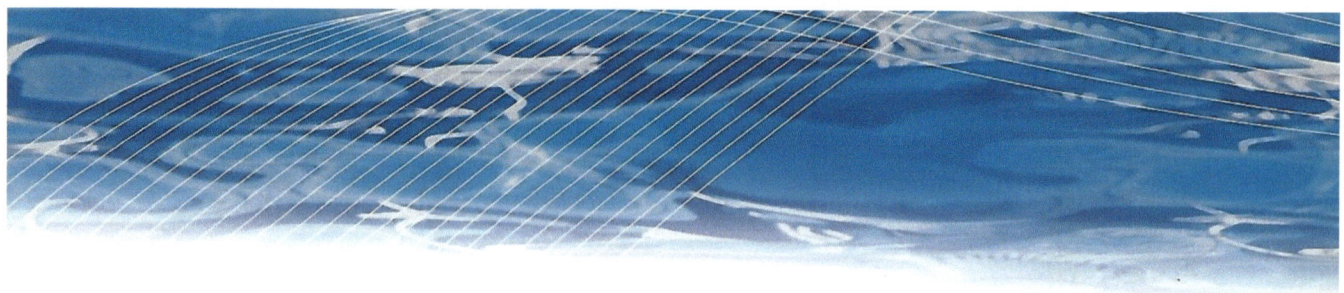

Better health from better water – THE Ionizer Plus®

Are you overly acidic?

Normal, healthy body functioning has extremely specific pH requirements. Arterial blood, for instance, has a pH between 7.35 and 7.45. Though the body utilizes a buffering mechanism to maintain a specific pH, this buffering mechanism can be stretched beyond its capacity by life's many sources of acidity. When the blood pH chronically sits toward the acidic side of this range, research shows this has a slow but steady negative impact on health[1].

Chronic disease, diet, lifestyle, stress, antibiotics, toxicity and aging all lead to an increasingly acidic shift within the body. Though our bodies can excrete much of this acidity, a kidney cannot excrete urine with a pH lower than 5 without significantly damaging the genitourinary tract. A can of cola has a pH between 2.8 and 3.2. To dilute a 12 ounce can of cola to a pH of 5, an additional 33 liters of urine would be required. Obviously this is not possible, so the body excretes some of its mineral supply to neutralize the acid. We are virtually bombarded by sources of acidity. Excess protein and fat in the diet, for example, are very common to the modern lifestyle and are a substantial source of acidity. Trying to avoid the many sources of acidity is virtually impossible and nearly every one of us, especially as we get older, is increasingly acidic.

Why is a body's increasingly acidic state bad?

This acidic state leads to a condition of malabsorption. Though a person's diet may include the needed nutrition, the body cannot properly absorb water and minerals. This results in mild but perpetual dehydration and mineral deficiency.

These problems inevitably lead to other, more serious chronic ailments. As the body's source of immediate buffer becomes stressed, the bones present an emergency source. Calcium is then robbed from the bones, ultimately resulting in decreased bone density and osteoporosis[2]. Besides affecting the bones, the digestive tract is also affected and is usually the first noticeable victim. Often starting with middle age, many people suffer from chronic heartburn, chronic indigestion, constipation, diarrhea, irritable bowel, or leaky gut.

Impaired nutrition also negatively affects the immune system. It is said that approximately 70% of our immune system resides in the gastrointestinal tract. A healthy digestive system is therefore critical to having a healthy immune system.

Are you overly acidic?
IF YOU HAVE TWO OR MORE OF THESE SYMPTOMS, YOU MAY BE SUFFERING FROM ACIDIC OVERLOAD. DRINKING IONIZED WATER CAN HELP TO RESTORE BALANCE TO YOUR BODY ELIMINATING THESE CHRONIC SIDE-EFFECTS.

: INDIGESTION	: CHRONIC DIARRHEA	: OSTEOPOROSIS
: POOR NUTRIENT ABSORPTION	: DEHYDRATION	: CHRONIC FATIGUE
: HEARTBURN	: POOR CIRCULATION	: FIBROMYALGIA
: NAUSEA	: MIGRAINES	: IRRITABLE BOWEL
: OBESITY	: ARTHRITIS	: LEAKY GUT
: CHRONIC CONSTIPATION	: HIGH BLOOD PRESSURE	

[1] L. Frassetto, R.C. Morris Jr., D.E. Sellmeyer, K. Todd, A. Sebastian, Diet, evolution and aging: The pathophysiologic effects of the post-agricultural inversion of the potassium-to-sodium and base-to-chloride ratios in the human diet, *Eur J Nutr* 40 :200 –213, 2001.

[2] Sherry A. Rogers, M.D., *Detoxify or Die* (www.prestigepublishing.com, 2002).

[3] K. Hanaoka, D. Sun, R. Lawrence, Y. Kamitani, G. Fernandez, *The mechanism of the enhanced antioxidant effects against superoxide anion radicals of reduced water produced by electrolysis*, Biophys Chem. 2004 Jan 1;107(1):71-82.

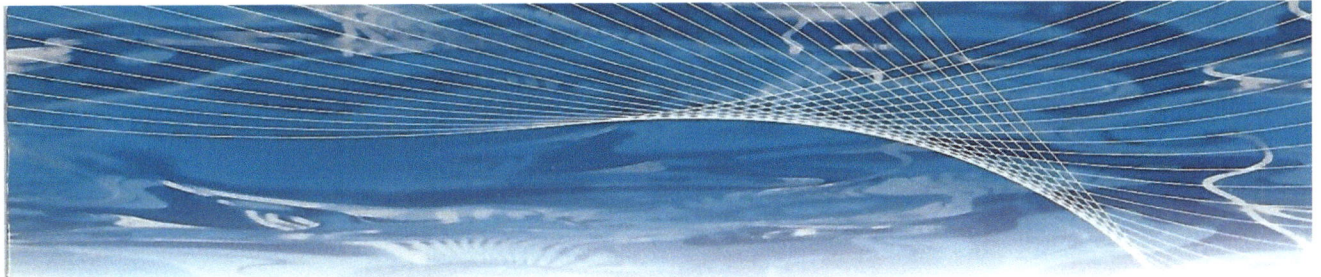

Better water for pennies a day

How can the Ionizer Plus® help?

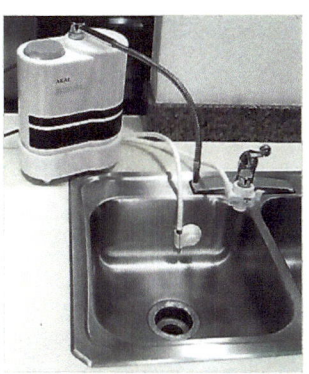

The solution is to return the body to a state of balance where it can heal itself of the other problems. The Ionizer Plus, through a process of electrolysis, concentrates minerals (calcium, magnesium, potassium) already present in your water. In the process of doing so, the minerals get split into the highly bioavailable ionic form and the resulting water is alkaline (has a pH greater than 7.0). The electrolysis process also reduces the surface tension of the water making the water itself more easily absorbed by the body.

Not only does this water help fight and reverse on-going acidity, but it also is a rich source of the very minerals robbed by acidity in the past.

What is electrolysis?

Electrolysis is the process that concentrates the minerals making the water alkaline. It accomplishes this by passing the water between two electrodes, one with a positive electric charge, the other with a negative electric charge. The minerals in the water then become reduced to their ionic form. Minerals such as calcium, magnesium and potassium have a positive charge and are attracted to the negatively charged electrode. This water, alkaline in nature, is then separated from the water attracted to the positively charged electrode.

The Ionizer Plus features Dura-Plat™ platinum coated titanium electrodes that are the best available anywhere. It is these electrodes that give our product the longest product design life of any water electrolyzer available – 12 to 14 years for an average family of four.

Enhances Antioxidants

Antioxidants are substances that protect cells and DNA from damage by unstable molecules called free radicals. Free radicals are molecules with incomplete electron shells that are highly reactive. They steal electrons from other molecules causing damage in the process. Free radicals are produced naturally during cellular metabolism and also result from exposure to environmental toxins and heavy metals.

Studies[3] have shown that the alkaline water resulting from electrolysis has the ability to improve the functioning of antioxidants. This means that consuming water from the Ionizer Plus enables antioxidants like vitamin C or even your body's natural antioxidants, such as superoxide dismutase (SOD), to neutralize more free radicals than otherwise would be possible. The negative ORP of the water has been shown to enhance the functioning of SOD further by helping to scavenge hydrogen peroxide, an intermediate yet still destructive oxygen species produced during SOD's reaction with free radicals.

30-Day Money Back Guarantee

We are so confident in our superior product that we guarantee your complete satisfaction. If you are not happy with your High Tech Health Ionizer Plus for any reason, you may return it any time within 30 days of receipt for a full refund (not including shipping).

CALL 1-800-794-5355 TODAY FOR A FREE ONE-ON-ONE CONSULTATION

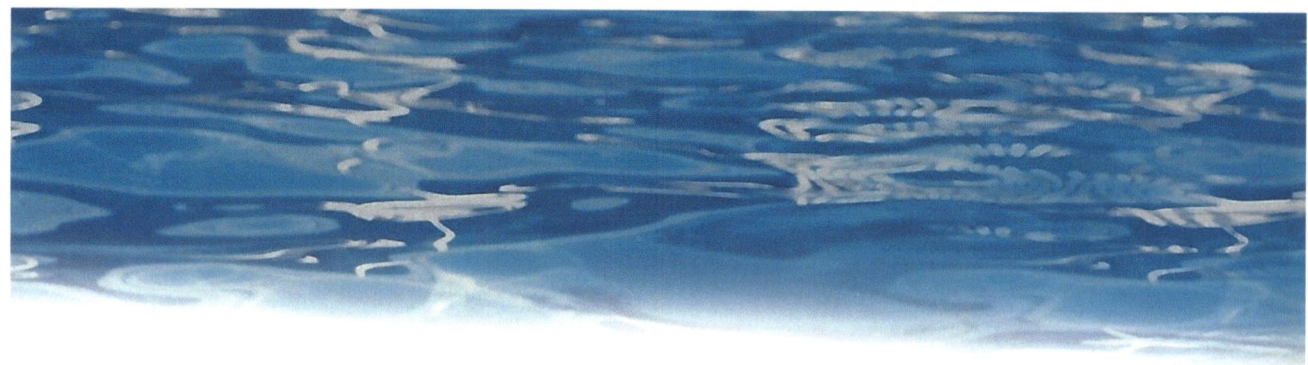

IONIZER PLUS® WATER ELECTROLYZER

INTELLIGENT DESIGN – GUARANTEED RESULTS – ATTRACTIVE – SIMPLE TO USE

Easy to change filter: Just open the cap, remove, and replace (filter lasts an average of one year for a family of four)

A single button changes the electrolysis mode from alkali, to acidic, to off (purifying).

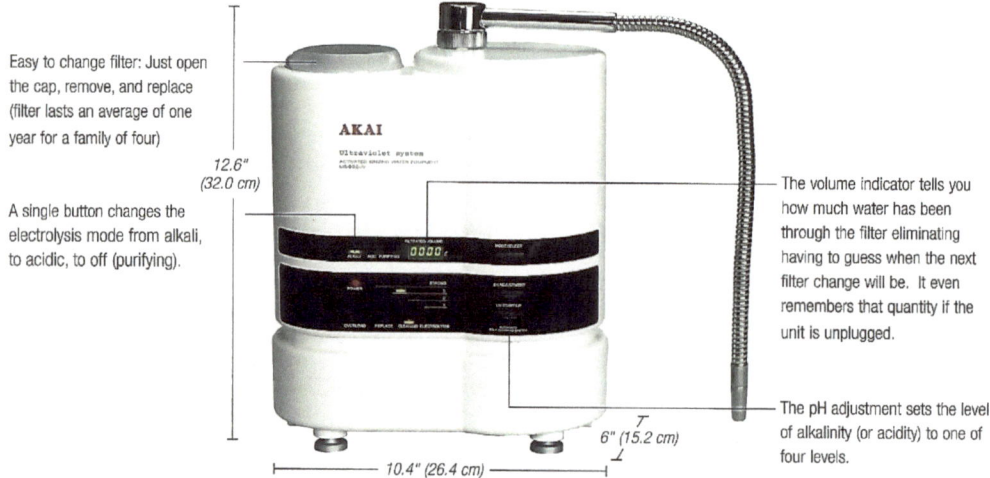

12.6"
(32.0 cm)

6" (15.2 cm)

10.4" (26.4 cm)

The volume indicator tells you how much water has been through the filter eliminating having to guess when the next filter change will be. It even remembers that quantity if the unit is unplugged.

The pH adjustment sets the level of alkalinity (or acidity) to one of four levels.

: GRANULAR ACTIVATED CARBON FILTER
Removes chlorine, and organic chemicals

: 0.1 MICRON MEMBRANE FILTER
Removes bacteria (and everything else larger than 0.1 micron)

: ELECTROLYSIS (WITH DURA-PLAT™ PLATINUM-COATED TITANIUM ELECTRODES)
Alkalizing
Mineralizing
Improved absorption (of both water and minerals)
Antioxidant enhancing

: ULTRAVIOLET (>8000 μW*sec/cm²)
Destroys virus

: SELF CLEANING

: A COMPUTER MONITORS THE FILTER'S LIFE, THE UV LIGHT, AND THE WATER PRESSURE TO ALERT YOU IF THERE WERE EVER ANY PROBLEM

AND IT EVEN COMES WITH A 30-DAY MONEY-BACK GUARANTEE.

BETTER HEALTH BEGINS WITH BETTER WATER.

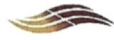 HIGH TECH HEALTH
INTERNATIONAL

4888 Pearl East Circle, Suite 202W
Boulder, Colorado 80301
Toll-free in North America 1-800-794-5355
Phone 303-413-8500 / Fax 303-449-9640
www.hightechhealth.com

 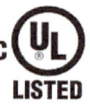
LISTED   LISTED

The statements contained herein have not been evaluated by the Food and Drug Administration. The Ionizer Plus is not intended to diagnose, treat, cure, or prevent any disease. Your results may vary. It is cesigned to work with potable water only.

CALL US TOLL-FREE TODAY AT 1-800-794-5355 FOR A PERSONALIZED CONSULTATION

One third of the water produced by the IONIZER PLUS WATER ELECTROLYZER is acidic water.

I personally use it to water my plants, for soaking my sprouts and spritzing my skin.

USES FOR ACIDIC WATER

Food: Wash your fruits, vegetables, and meats to effectively kill any bacteria.

Plant Care: Watering your plants and vegetables will promote growth and reduce fungus. Cut flowers will last longer in acidic water as well.

Cleaning: The acidic water is very effective for disinfecting, therefore it's great for cleaning counter tops, sinks, glass, floors, etc.

Antiseptic: Can be used as an antiseptic for abrasions, cuts, and healing as well as a mouthwash to assist in removing bacteria from your mouth. Just be sure to rinse again afterwards with alkaline water.

Skin care: The acidic water, used topically, penetrates the skin, kills any bacteria, hydrates the skin, and restores the natural pH. Splashing the acidic water on your face can improve the complexion of your skin without the use of chemicals. I like to splash the acidic water on my face right after cleansing. It's also great to put into a spray bottle and use as a toner. A light mist can set makeup beautifully as well. Make sure to dab the water specifically under the eyes, where skin is most permeable and ages the fastest. It's a great little "anti-aging" secret no one ever seems to mention! Men can use the acidic water as an aftershave. Any skincare products you apply after splashing the face with acidic water will help the product penetrate deeper & work that much better.

It can also relieve dry and itchy skin, and expedite the healing process of cuts, scrapes, insect bites, rashes, sunburns, athlete's foot, nail fungus, blisters, acne, psoriasis, and even poison ivy irritation.

Hair Care: After you have shampooed your hair, pour the acidic water slowly over your head. It will penetrate your hair like a conditioner, making your hair healthier, slightly thicker, and provide a natural shine without using chemical products. It's also effective for addressing hair loss, dandruff or scalp irritation.

Enjoy these suggested uses for the acidic ionized water!

Call (800) 794-5355 toll free to speak with any High Tech Health Product Specialist to receive a substantial discount off this wonderful product!
Be sure to mention the name Christine Lauren or this book's title Health Made Simple! for your discount.

I received this letter in response to a request for information regarding the Kangen water purifier:

Ionizer Plus vs. Kangen

1. Kangen uses additives in their water such as calcium sulphite (calcium salt) and sodium hypochloride (bleach). They add these chemicals to help their units produce a higher pH than it would otherwise. Calcium sulphite is not good for anyone with heart or hypertension problems. It is not only a health hazard but additives break down the platinum coating on the electrolysis plates, decreasing the life of the Kangen product.

2. Their five-year-old technology costs the consumer approximately $3,980 for one machine. The Ionizer Plus is substantially less expensive; especially when the available discount is applied. Kangen is a multi-level company, which accounts for their mark up.

Ionizer Plus compared to Kangen:

The Ionizer Plus requires only 2 electrolysis plates due to its power efficiency, which is 200 watts and has Dura-Plat Platinum coated Titanium Electrodes. Kangen requires multiple plates to compensate for the lower power efficiency, which can result in long term corrosion and mineral deposit build up forcing the machine to stop working.

High Tech Health is the only company that offers an optional cleaning cartridge that is a natural citric acid that will dissolve any mineral deposit that has built up on the interior of the machine extending the life of the machine. Our machine also has a low-dose ultraviolet light that no other machine has including Kangen. The UV light removes ail viruses from your water. The carbon portion of our filter filters out all chlorine and chemicals along with our hollow-fiber membrane filter, which filters out anything larger than 0.1 microns. This includes all bacteria, such as e.coli, giardia, and crypto-sporidium. The water is then treated with a direct current creating electrolysis, the splitting of oxygen and hydrogen, which concentrates the minerals (calcium, magnesium and potassium) already present in your water.

Keep in mind also that Enagic, the multi-level marketing company that sells the Kangen machine, has no UV light, offers only 3 alkaline settings, has multiple plates due to low power efficiency, and most importantly, their filters use Calcium Sulfite ($CaSO_3$), which is **calcium salt that is added to every glass of water that you drink.** Over time this salt causes heavy build up on their multiple plates and can cause serious damage to the machine and to their clients' health. Their machine also adds Sodium Hypo-Chlorite to the reservoir of their machine (which is similar to bleach) and this forces the electrolysis to produce extreme pH levels, which is used for their marketing strategies regarding extreme cleaning.

Call (800) 794-5355 toll free to speak with any High Tech Health Product Specialist to receive a substantial discount off this wonderful product!
Be sure to mention the name Christine Lauren or this book's title Health Made Simple! for your discount.

I hope the following information helps you understand the cause of some of the things you may be struggling with...

MAINTENANCE OF THE BODY'S pH

Your body regulates its pH just like it regulates its temperature. In doing so, it will even create stress on other tissues or body systems if necessary to maintain its proper pH.

Since your blood MUST maintain a very narrow pH range of 7.365 to 7.40, **your body will do all sorts of things in order to deal with excess acidity.**

It will **flush excess acids into fat cells** (which is **why you can't seem to lose those extra pounds**...the fat is protecting internal organs from the acids).

Or, perhaps, it will **leach calcium** (an alkaline mineral) from your bones in order to neutralize acids.

Your body will also **stress tissues by flushing acids into them** (as is the case with gout) because it cannot dump these acids into the bloodstream (which must remain alkaline or you would die).

When the pH of our bodies becomes too acidic, we may experience low energy, fatigue, excess weight, poor digestion, aches and pains, and even more serious disorders.

The body becomes imbalanced and overly acidic primarily as a result of three things:

1. **Ingesting acids.** Eating too many acidifying foods creates an **acid ash** in the body. These acids can overload your body's ability to neutralize them.

2. **Creation of acids.** An acidic environment is a breeding ground for **toxic microforms.** Since these organisms are living, they steal your nutrients, and create **acidic toxins.**

3. **Improper elimination of acids.** The body uses many systems in order to buffer acids, including fat, breath and mineral reserves. When the body's buffering systems become compromised, excess acids build up.

Be encouraged that there is hope that all of these factors can be corrected through the four simple basic steps and habits presented in this book. When all four building blocks are used together they potentially correct the root of the dilemmas we have with our health, working together to set us free to function as lovingly designed ... with vibrant health and energy.

This is the water therapy method mentioned previously that I follow:

Water Therapy

*This information is included for educational purposes only
and has not been verified through documented studies.*

Popular in Japan and India.

Water Therapy - Method of Treatment

1. As you wake up in the morning before brushing teeth, drink **two 16-ounce glasses of water.**
2. Do not eat or drink anything for 45 minutes.
3. After 45 minutes, you may eat and drink as normal.
4. If unable to drink all of the water at the outset you may commence by taking a little water and gradually increase it to the recommended amount.

Also, do not drink any alcoholic beverages the previous evening.

Benefits of Water Therapy

Relief from stress, weight loss, glowing skin, feeling fresh and energetic throughout the day and good digestion are some of the major benefits of water therapy.

Japanese Medical Society Proves Its Value

A Japanese medical society (not known which one specifically) has found it profoundly helped the following diseases:

- Headache
- Body Ache
- Heart System
- Arthritis
- Rapid Heart Beat
- Epilepsy
- Excess fat
- Bronchitis
- Asthma
- TB
- Meningitis

- Kidney and Urinary diseases
- Vomiting
- Gastritis
- Diarrhea
- Piles (hemorrhoids)
- Diabetes
- Constipation
- Eye Diseases
- Menstrual Disorders
- Ear Nose Throat Diseases

The following list gives the number of days of treatment they have found to cure main diseases:

1. High Blood Pressure - 30 days
2. Gastric - 10 days
3. Diabetes - 30 days
4. Constipation - 10 days
5. Tuberculosis – 90 days
6. Arthritis patients need to be on this regimen for only three days.

This treatment method has **no side effects,** however at the commencement of treatment you may have to urinate more.

How does pure water help the body?

This method purifies the human body.

Water renders the colon more effective by enabling it to form fresh new blood, known in medical terms as hemopoiesis.

This purification process activates the mucosal folds of the colon and intestines because fresh, the mucosal fold produces new blood.

When the colon is cleansed then the nutrients of the food taken several times a day will be absorbed and by the action of the mucosal folds they are turned into fresh blood.
End of Japanese water therapy information

In my opinion this is significant because the blood is all-important in curing ailments and restoring health. "The life is in the blood", according to the Bible in Leviticus 17:11.

In addition, I received the following information from a friend regarding the benefits of drinking water during different times of the day: Again, this information is for educational purposes only.

Heart Attack & Water

Here's something I didn't know! I asked my doctor why people urinate so much at night.

Answer from my cardiac doctor:
Gravity holds water in the lower part of your body when you are upright (legs swell). When you lie down the legs and feet are level with the kidneys and then the kidneys can remove water from the body more easily. I knew you needed water to help flush the toxins out of your body, but this was news to me.

Also, drinking water at a certain time maximizes its effectiveness in the body:
2 glasses of water after waking up– *helps activate internal organs*
1 glass of water 30 minutes before a meal- *helps digestion*
1 glass of water before taking a bath- *helps lower blood pressure*
1 glass of water before going to bed– *avoids stroke or heart attack*

He also told me that water at bedtime would also help prevent nighttime leg cramps because your leg muscles are seeking hydration when they cramp and wake you up with a "Charlie horse".

This is why water therapy is recommended to be added to your daily routine.

Important note from the author: *Please note this theory has not been proven clinically. However, I have been on this water therapy regime for quite a few months. I have been drinking two 16-ounce glasses of water upon waking up and have not been sick once since starting! I wish good health to you with Water Therapy!*

STEP TWO: GREEN SUPER FOOD

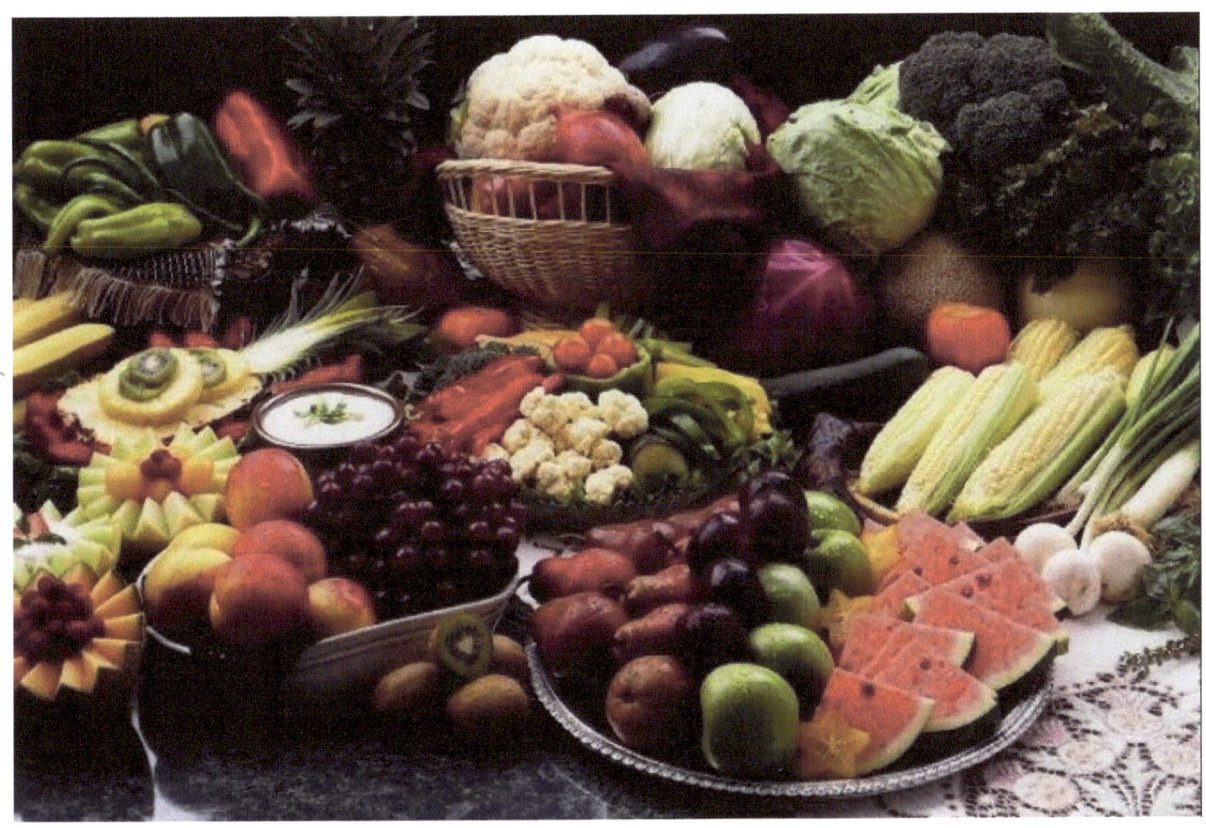

In a perfect world we would choose to sit down to this banquet every day!

But we don't live in a perfect world. **So how do we get food of this quality on a daily basis and in a way that is not time consuming?** I am eternally grateful that in 1985 I received a fluorescent green tri-fold from a friend I went to school with that told me about Barley Green, now called **Barley-Life.** Barley Life is food of the highest possible quality. Its quality is so high it is considered a super food.

If it weren't for Barley-Life I am certain I would be in chronic neck pain. Barley Life is barley grass grown to about ten or twelve inches high that is cut, juiced and then the juice is dried at a low temperature so that it maintains the vital nutrients and live enzymes that have been life changing for me. After being dried it is available in a powder form or a capsule.

I take two tablespoons of it in powder form in water every day and I no longer have joint pain, allergies or fibromyalgia. Even more spectacular is that I don't have chronic neck pain. If I go a week without it, my neck begins to ache because it was broken at birth, which inflicted nerve damage.

Why I love Barley-Life

It is alive! It's processed at a low temperature to protect the enzymes and other nutrients in it. It is predigested so it goes directly into the bloodstream. It does a wonderful job of helping the body to have a healthy alkaline pH.

My Story:

I first learned about Barley-Life (then called Barley Green) in 1985 when a friend from high school gave me a bright green tri-fold about it. John had a Barley Green belt that he kept cinching in as he took Barley Green. Because it met his nutritional needs, he naturally lost weight. He didn't change his primarily pizza diet. His belt went in about a foot.

I attended a meeting with him and clearly remember a young man in his 30s who was there with his father. The son had had a tumor at the base of his neck. The tumor was eradicated with radiation but he was left with headaches that no narcotic painkiller could touch. His dad suggested he try Barley Green. He took it for a week. After a week, his headaches had gone away. Then the headaches came back. His dad asked him if he were drinking anything hot after he took the Barley Green to which he said he had been. He learned to wait half an hour before drinking anything hot and his headaches went away again. The hot liquid affects the live enzymes in the Barley Green.

I personally have a vertebra in my neck (top one) that is "out like a scout" according to a chiropractor I visited. He said he wouldn't even touch my neck unless I did 6 months of exercise to strengthen it. He also pointed out in the x-ray that my neck had been broken.

This was not surprising since I was a blue baby strangled in the birthing process. As long as I faithfully take 2 tablespoons of Barley-Life a day I am pain free. I make sure I don't run out because in less than a week my neck starts aching.

Before Barley-Life, I had severe allergies and joint pain to the point that I couldn't go into certain stores because all the synthetics in them made me sick. I guess you would say I was environmentally sensitive. I also had stress related fibromyalgia. I have lived in beautiful South Carolina since 2002. I know people here who suffer with allergies. **I credit Barley- Life with the fact that I have no allergies, no joint pain, no fibromyalgia and no neck ache.**

In 1995 my dad had bone cancer. I told him about Barley-Life and he began taking it along with some other health products. In one week he went from not being able to get out of his chair to walking around the block with me. In addition, my mother had colon cancer before I learned about Barley-Life. For that reason I also take Barley-Life as what I consider to be a good preventive measure since it helps keep the pH alkaline.

Barley-Life has been my ace in the hole. I would never be without it. My neck would be talking to me in short order with pain if I didn't take it!

Following is the green brochure I received in 1985.

CAPTURE YOUR DREAM
AND FEEL THE DIFFERENCE WITH
BARLEY GREEN

Any **DREAM** or **GOAL** of increased health, wealth and happiness requires planning, effort, and more energy. In addition to more energy —

People using Barley Green are Reporting Benefits such as —

Less Sleep Required

More Stamina & Energy

High Blood Pressure Reduced

Freedom From Pain Pills

Relief Of Stomach-Ache And Stomach Ulcer

Reduced Pain & Inflammation Of Arthritis

Solved Acne Problems

Improved Regularity

Weight Loss Made Easier

"Barley Grass tastes something like tea and it's one of the most incredible products of this decade! It improves Stamina, Sexual energy, Clarity of thought and reduces addiction to things that are bad for you. It also improves the texture of skin and heals the dryness associated with aging" Dr. Howard Lutz, Director of the Institute for Preventive Medicine, Washington D.C.

"Arthritic pain almost gone, no more drugs, better complexion, praise the Lord for Barley Green." Dixie Mudd, Kent, Wa.

"Was on my death bed with lymphoma cancer, 3 months on B.G. and in total remission. 5 years super health, no recurrence." Rosie Sturm, Eagle, Id

"Improved stamina and increased sense of well being." / "As a cosmetologist standing many hours, much more energy." Emery & Dorothy Tedrick, Edmonds, Wa.

"Relief from stress is spelled BARLEY GREEN. " Julie Jimenez, Kent, Wa.

"Sinuses & allergies greatly improved. Increased energy & stamina." Glen & Inez Tweet, Seattle, Wa.

"Arthritic pain & headaches gone in less than a week, no recurrence." Pam Smith, Fedral Way, Wa.

"Facial skin cancer & growths have healed & disappeared, athlete's foot gone." Ken Abendroth, Seattle, Wa.

"Hypoglycemic symptoms gone. 3 hours more productivity a day." Ginger Carollo, Auburn, Wa.

"More energy, less sleep." / "If I miss my B.G., my mother's milk doesn't satisfy baby." Ed & Heidi Kendall, Kent, Wa.

"Regained the energy of a teenager without the acne." Don Failla, Romona, Ca. Lecturer, author, MLM expert.

"Watched the cancer disappear in our dog's ear. Two years later no recurrence." Al & Sharon Gilleck, Stanwood, Wa.

"Never felt so good!" Dennis & Mary L. Goldner, Tacoma, Wa.

"Addiction to cigarettes gone." / "Blood count normal in only 4 months after 1 & 1½ years chemotherapy & radiation, PTL." Doug & June Bushaw, Fed. way, Wa.

"Lower blood pressure, after 5 wks. Relief from edema." / "Night vision 100% better 4 days, weight loss easier." Joe & Lory Gomez, Kent, Wa.

"The most amazing and fantastic product I've ever run into for health, energy and stamina" Dr. Richard You, Physician and trainer for past U.S. Olympic teams.

"Arthritic pain had been encouraging early retirement. Now with B.G. many years of productivity left." Dale Telford, Fed. Way, Wa.

We make no "healing claims" for Barley Green. It balances the body. B.G. delivers potent levels of nutrition and live enzymes on the cellular level, which enhances energy. This also allows the immune system to attack disease, thus helping the body to heal itself.

THE ULTIMATE BALANCE
of
LIVING LIQUID NUTRITION!
Not just another vitamin & mineral supplement

DR. YOSHIHIDI HAGIWARA'S discovery of BARLEY GREEN is the result of 13 years of intensive research looking for the ultimate & broadest spectrum of nutrition for the human cell. Barley Green is a concentrated juice which is dehydrated to a powder at low temperatures, allowing the enzymes to remain alive. There are no indigestible substances. All the nutrients, chlorophyll, enzymes, vitamins, and minerals are balanced by nature and readily assimilable being absorbed directly through the cell membranes in the mouth, throat, stomach and digestive tract. Because of Barley Green's concentrated potency, small amounts are generally sufficient for an individual to experience the results of super nutrition, within a matter of days. Typical usage includes 3 servings daily ranging from ½ to 2 grams per serving. (Most start with ½ gram per serving) 2 grams is approximately 1 teaspoon. Mixed with 6 oz. of cold water, Barley Green has a mild yet stimulating taste of freshly-cut barley leaves. Some prefer to mix B.G. with vegetable, grape, apple, or orange juice. Some examples of B.G.'s SUPER NUTRITION ARE:

OVER 250 TIMES THE VITAMIN A IN LETTUCE
OVER 25 TIMES THE POTASSIUM IN BANANAS
OVER 11 TIMES THE CALCIUM IN COWS' MILK
OVER 11 TIMES THE IRON IN CELERY
OVER 7 TIMES THE VITAMIN C IN ORANGES
OVER 10 TIMES THE VITAMIN B1 IN SPINACH
OVER 23 TIMES THE BIOTIN IN COWS' MILK
2000 MICROGRAMS OF LIVE S.O.D. IN EACH
2 -GRAM SERVING

MORE BARLEY GREEN REPORTS

"Shopping for wheelchair (arthritis), in 2 weeks walking 2 miles." Ruth Andrews, Ballard, Wa.

"Two hours less sleep a night. Puts me to work sooner with more energy. Gives me more time for my work and my family." Ray Mudd, Kent, Wa.

"Was addicted to antacids. Gastric distress eliminated with B.G." Del Johnson, Fed. Way, Wa.

"More vitality, stamina," / "Solution to air pollution." Steve & Naomi O'Connor, Renton, Wa.

(Vertical letters along column:)
R E V E R S I N G   T H E   A G I N G   P R O C E S S

All joints are sealed cavities filled with a lubricant cushion called synovial fluid. In normal joint function, synovial fluid or "joint oil" is kept in a healthy condition by S.O.D. — CATALASE ENZYME COMPLEX. These "body produced" enzymes clean impurities called "free radicals" from the "joint oil" or synovial fluid keeping the joint properly lubricated and allowing free movement. Cellular underproduction of S.O.D. — CATALASE ENZYME COMPLEX, due to diet, stress, heavy exercise, or aging allows these gritty toxins or "free radicals" to accumulate in the joint causing friction, heat, swelling and eventual damage to the joint itself.

S.O.D. — CATALASE ENZYME COMPLEX in proper amounts provides the body with nutritional tools to remove the impurities from synovial fluid in a natural way allowing proper lubrication and free movement to return.

SOD is a live protein enzyme that deactivates free radicals. A free radical is an extremely unstable oxygen molecule, which like an uncontrolled projectile inflicts damage to many substances in our bodies. Dr. Milton Fried, M.D. says that the damage inflicted by these free radicals shows up as aging of the body and disease. Dr. Fried also says, "If we can increase the SOD in the cells, we may have THE FOUNTAIN OF YOUTH MAN HAS SEARCHED FOR FOR GENERATIONS." In an article by Ti Nesi, in the 3/18/80 issue of National Enquirer. There is no cure for aging; nothing can prevent aging from taking place — but scientists now believe that perhaps S.O.D. delays it.
(Science Digest, August, 1982).

BEE PROPOLIS GIVES CELL PROTECTION

Propolis is a resinous substance collected by bees from the sap and leaf buds of trees. Propolis is used in the bee hive as a sealing agent. Because of the strong antibacterial, antiviral and antifungal properties of Propolis, it is said that the interior of a honey bee hive is one of the most sterile environments in nature.

Propolis has been shown to be effective in greatly reducing susceptibility to and in speeding the recovery from colds, upper respiratory infections and influenza. A 1981 Russian study concluded Propolis was even effective against certain strains of bacteria which have become resistant to tetracycline and erythromycin drugs.

Excerpts of Dr. Hagiwara's speech

Madison Square Garden, N.Y., N.Y.

"Thank you, Mr. Chairman, and Ladies and Gentlemen!! It is great honor for me to be given this opportunity to talk to you about "How to attain and maintain good health". As I was introduced to you, my name is YOSHIHIDE HAGIWARA, and I am a Medical Doctor. I am one of the promoters of "Health Campaign in Japan". I am now going to talk about "How to enjoy Good Health, Rejuvenation, and Longevity". I am going to talk about "Food".

Our foods contain lots of chemical substances, and manufactured foodstuffs are lacking in vitamins, minerals and necessary enzymes. Water is polluted with many chemicals and heavy metals; air is polluted with smog which contains petroleum by-products. Furthermore, in mass-production of processed foods in factories, colorants, preservatives and antioxidants are used to improve their appearance and preserve them. Moreover, the processed foods contain less vitamins and minerals than natural foods.

Now that our diet is going to lack in raw vegetables, I have invented "young green barley juice powder" to make up for the shortage of raw vegetables. A spoonful of "young barley juice powder" contains equivalent extracts of two heads of lettuce or one head of cabbage.

In this fresh and raw "young green juice powder", there are enzymes almost similar to those existing in the body cells of man. The enzymes aid in our digestion and counteract poisons. For example, Superoxide dismutase, recently a topic as an effective enzyme for its preventive action against cellular aging, collagen diseases and leukemia.

We have discovered that this "Young green barley juice powder" contains elements which can prevent cancer and counteract mutations.

It has come to be known that char in broiled fish and meat contains Try P-1 and Try P-2 which include 20,000 times as strong carcinogenicity as that of 3, 4 benzpyrene of tobacco which will cause lung cancers.

However, our "young green barley juice powder" prevents cancer by decomposing all these elements. 17 years ago, the FDA announced that 3, 4 benzpyrene causes lung cancer, however last year it was made public at the Japan Pharmaceutical Society that this "young green barley juice" greatly reduces the risk and neutralizes the poisonous effects of 3, 4 benzpyrene.

70% of carcinogens are nitric compounds, which are believed to be the decomposition products of petroleum products. The components of this "young green barley juice powder" have been proved to be antidote and counteract the poisonous compounds.

"Young green barley juice powder" counteracts inflammation. Our experiments have proven that this anti-inflammatory substance is superior to cortizone or steroid and phenylbutazone. What's more, this "green barley juice powder" has no side effects.

At the 101st conference of Japan Pharmaceutical Society, Dr. YASUO HOTTA of the University of California, together with us, reported that this "young green barley juice powder" has restorative power of DNA. It will be proved in the near future that this "young green barley juice powder" will be used as a preventive means against cancer.

Now, Ladies and Gentlemen, we desire "rejuvenating power" that will make us young and vigorous again in nature and appearance. The fair sex, girls, and women desire for "young and fresh, soft, beautiful skin". By drinking this "young green barley juice" everyday, they can keep their skin young, fresh, soft and beautiful.

As I have already stated, our "young green barley juice" with its vitamins and minerals, can counteract carcinogens, restore ulcer injured cells, appease inflammation and restore damaged DNA. By our research it has come to be known that this "young juice powder" will bring about the "gospel" of health.

Thank you!! God bless you all !!

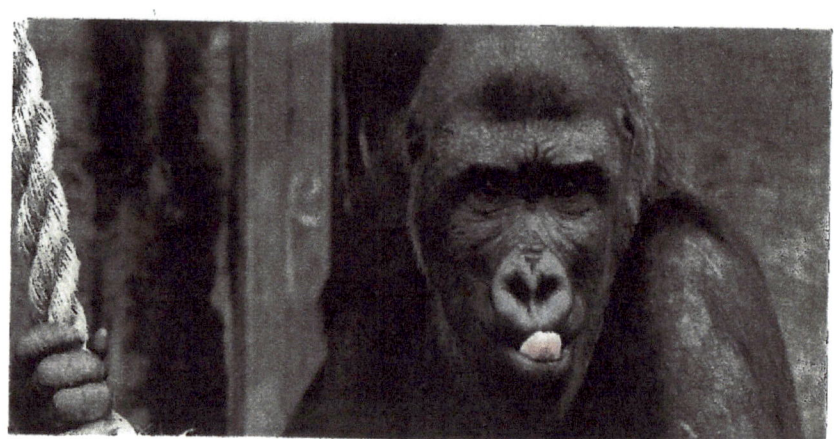

Hmm, let's think about it...how strong is a silverback gorilla compared to a human?

Some say **10 times stronger**. Though never measured, these animals have been observed to almost casually bend and snap tempered steel bars (2 inches thick) and giant bamboo stalks. This suggests that the gorilla has the muscle power of between 8-15 men--possibly more!

Jersey Zoo's Jambo was observed hanging from one arm (he was over 400 lbs) while methodically ripping over 200 feet of inner ceiling planks from the roof of the new gorilla house with his other arm (the planks were securely screwed and nailed), simply because he didn't like them.

No other animal outside of the great apes has such an amazing combination of strength and dexterity.

Where do they get their strength? They are mainly vegetarian, eating fruits, leaves, and shoots. Insects make up 1-2% of their diet.

Why would their diet of greens produce such strength?

❶ Greens are direct conduits of the sun's energy. This energy goes directly into their bloodstream, the "river of life".

❷ Greens also are highly alkaline-forming in the body, important because disease cannot thrive in an alkaline environment. Ever seen a gorilla blowing his nose?

❸ Per ounce, greens provide a lot more protein than meat.

So it's no wonder that the strongest and biggest animals live on grass and green leaves!

Look at the elephant!

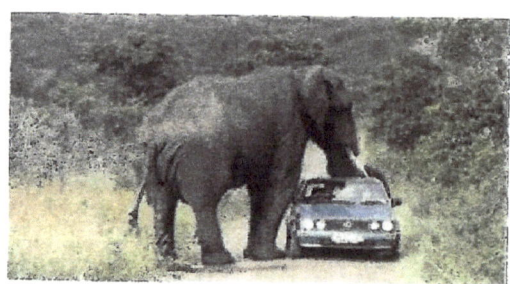

By far one of the largest, strongest and smartest mammals on the planet with one of the longest life spans- 69 years!
And the elephant eats nothing but grass!

Because people are seeking new understanding and solutions to their health dilemmas, it's a good thing that AIM is a multi-level company that will reimburse you for your efforts if you choose to use and share this great product.

You can order it by calling the The A.I.M. Companies in Nampa, Idaho at 800-456-2462 (MST). **Just give them my I.D. number 39706 as your sponsor. Best price for you is if you sign up as a member to purchase at wholesale. $100 in product waives the $20 membership fee. Barley-Life (12.7 oz. family size) is $48 member (wholesale) price. $62.50 retail. Shipping fees are added to all orders.**

When asked if you want to become a **member to purchase at wholesale** *I would suggest saying "yes" because of these benefits:*

1. *You receive an average of* **30% savings** *on products purchased*

2. *You can* **sign people up** *to purchase product under your ID number*

3. *You will receive a* **monthly magazine with your money order**

4. *You will have the opportunity to participate in and benefit from AIM's* **compensation plan.**

When you become a wholesale member there is **no obligation** *to purchase a certain amount of product per month. In addition you will receive your own ID number.*

OR

You also have the option of purchasing as a **retail customer**.

TIPS ON TAKING BARLEY LIFE

Because Barley Life is a live food it contains live enzymes. Mix it in a shaker or blender in cold or room temperature water or juice but not into a hot liquid. Be sure to **wait at least half an hour** after taking it before drinking anything hot because the heat will kill the live enzymes.

I suggest you **work up gradually** to taking 2 tablespoons per day. Nine caplets equal one tablespoon if you prefer caplets.

I've heard of people who took it at night and it gave them so much energy they couldn't go to sleep so it's better to **take it in the morning**.

Also, once you have blended it up, **drink it right away**. The enzymes will deteriorate if they are left sitting in a glass.

I would also suggest that you **take it consistently for three months**. This seems to be a physiological turn- around time.

Best wishes!

BOTH WATER AND EXCELLENT NUTRITION CONTRIBUTE TO A HEALTHY COLON

It really is true that health starts in the colon!

The diagram of the large intestine (colon) on the following page shows which area of the colon absorbs nutrients for various parts of the body. Notice in the diagram that it systematically absorbs nutrients from the head down through the entire body. If the colon is not cleaned out, the body starves regardless of the amount of food consumed because it can easily become impacted and dysfunctional especially when processed foods are consumed.

Truly, our Creator fearfully and wonderfully makes us!

Herbal Fiberblend is one of the first two products made available from The AIM Companies. The other product is Barley-Life, which you were just recently made aware of. I love Herbal Fiberblend because it not only cleans out the colon but the other organs in our bodies as well. It has herbs in it, including those that include those that kill or expel parasites. I believe it can also enable the body to get rid of the *black rope that is caused by eating margarine. Margarine is made from hydrogenated oil and cannot be digested. It is a health hazard.*

I still take Herbal Fiberblend and it is still available from AIM. To order Herbal Fiberblend, call The AIM Companies at 800-456-2462 and sign up as a member so that you will have your own personal ID number. That gives you the benefit of a *30% average discount*, and membership is FREE with a minimum order of $100. Be sure to provide my sponsor ID number 39706 when you sign up. You will receive a *monthly magazine with your money order*. You will also have the opportunity to participate in and benefit from AIM's *compensation plan*. When you become a wholesale member there is *no obligation* to purchase a certain amount of product per month. In addition you will receive your own ID number.

Herbal Fiberblend is $35 member (wholesale) price, $45.50 retail. Shipping fees are added to all orders.

This diagram of the colon clearly demonstrates the truth of the Biblical principle to do all things decently and in order *1 Corinthians 14: 40.*
Notice that nutrients are sequentially absorbed in the colon from the top of the head to the tip of the toes.
Just as in the Body of Christ, every part of the body is essential and worthy of care and nourishment.
Without a doubt, we are fearfully and wonderfully made!

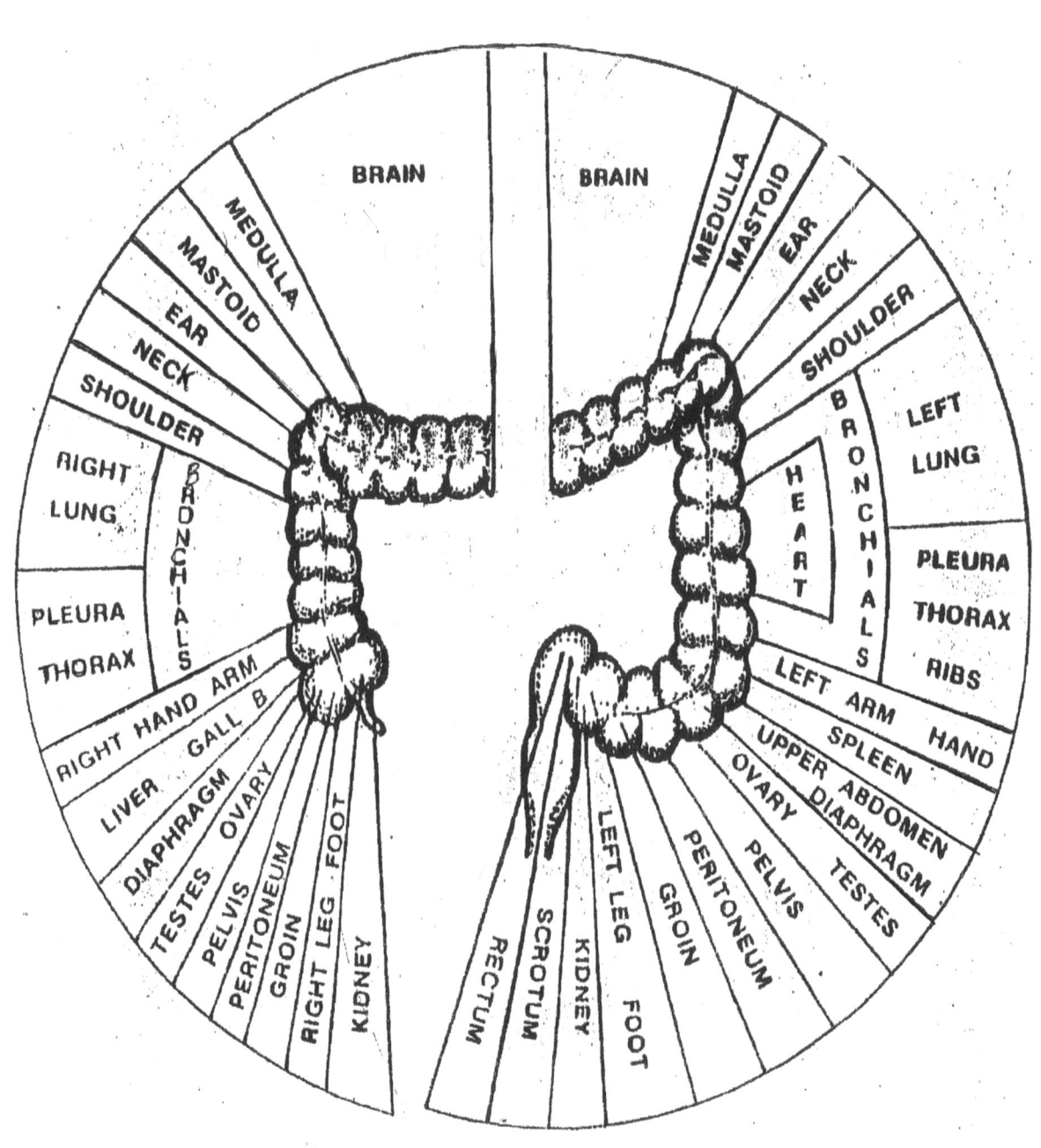

STEP THREE: HIMALAYAN SALT

You might be saying to yourself that your doctor told you to steer clear of salt, and for a very good reason explained more fully in the following four pages.

Common table salt is a nightmare for the human body. It is heated to over **1,200** degrees F., which alters its natural chemical structure. But even more disastrous is that it contains an anti-caking agent and **it is this anti-caking agent that goes into the blood vessels and causes high blood pressure, not the salt itself.**

Like a lot of us, I bought all sorts of bottles of vitamins and minerals trying to meet the needs of my body. Then an absolutely wonderful solution came my way. I learned about salt, wonderful Himalayan salt!

Salt is one of the most wonderful gifts from God. Obviously it's meant to be consumed because if not, we wouldn't have taste buds for salt. It's essential for correct bodily functions. **Himalayan salt contains the 84 trace elements and minerals that are also in our bloodstream.** I'm sure you've visited people in the hospital being given IVs of saline (salt) solution. This is to replenish minerals and restore bodily fluids if dehydrated.

I'm also impressed that these 84 trace elements and minerals are related to one another in proper proportion. No more having to figure it out! No more saying, "OK. I need two of these and one of these and have to take them after I eat."

Since I've begun putting Himalayan salt into the water I drink every day, I've stopped having the muscle cramps that I used to get at night. In the evening I drink a glass of water with ½ tsp. of Himalayan salt in it.

It's amazing to me that this salt is virtually the same as our blood. The Bible declares that the life is in the blood. I consider Himalayan salt to be an amazing blood tonic.

I am also amazed that these 84 elements are arranged in perfect quantity and relationship to one another. Who but an amazing Creator God could do something like that? So no more having cupboards full of vitamins and minerals that demand taking one with two after meals. That complexity is solved with wonderful Himalayan salt.

And, in-addition, so many of our foods are not grown in mineral rich soils, so they are depleted. before they even arrive at the grocery store. This salt is perpetually a source of what we need for our health, not dependent as plant life is on the quality of soil, how long it has been in a container box aboard a ship or how it may have been genetically altered by man.

Today's common table salt has nothing in common with natural salt.

Common table salt is **heated** to over 1,200 degrees Fahrenheit, which alters the natural chemical structure of the salt.

AND

It contains an **anti-caking agent**, which goes into the blood vessels and *this agent is what causes high blood pressure, not the salt itself*.

This anti-caking agent is sodium ferro cyanide is a chemical additive known as E 535 in the EU. Considered "not especially toxic" it is added to road and food grade salt as an anti-caking agent.

When combined with iron, it converts to a deep blue pigment called Prussian blue. In photography it is used for bleaching, toning and fixing. It is produced industrially from hydrogen cyanide, ferrous chloride and calcium hydroxide. *(Information from Wikipedia)*

Unlike natural salt, table salt has no life and requires great energy from our bodies to even partially metabolize it.

Below is common table salt at 400X magnification:

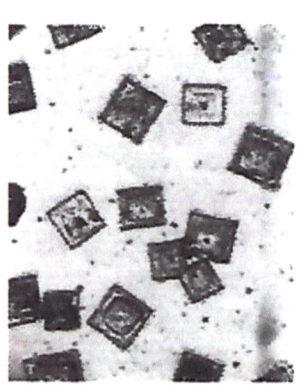

Salt, wonderful natural salt!

Natural salt, by contrast, is dynamic and contains powerful, life building forces for the organs and nervous system.

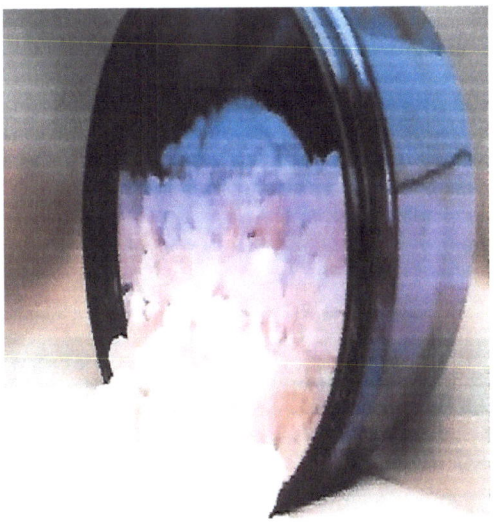

Enlarged to 400x magnification below

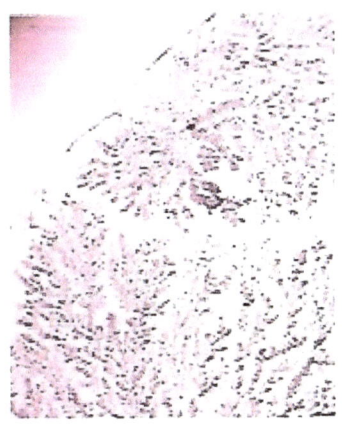

This picture shows a delicate, living structure, which is an excellent food source. Its delicate branching exhibits its vitality.

Because this natural crystal contains all the elements that exist on earth, our body consists of the same elements as water and salt.

Even the ratio of concentration of salt in our blood equals that of water from the ocean.

Natural salt contains the 84 elements found in our blood stream.

Natural salt has been used in emergency surgery on animals successfully as a replacement for blood.

When ingested, this wonderful salt stimulates intestinal activity, which stimulates metabolism and digestion.

Electrolytes are created which improve the body's conductivity and stimulate the circulation. Salt allows the current to flow thus contributing to health of the heart and other organs.

This is comparable to a battery, which uses copper and zinc to conduct electricity.

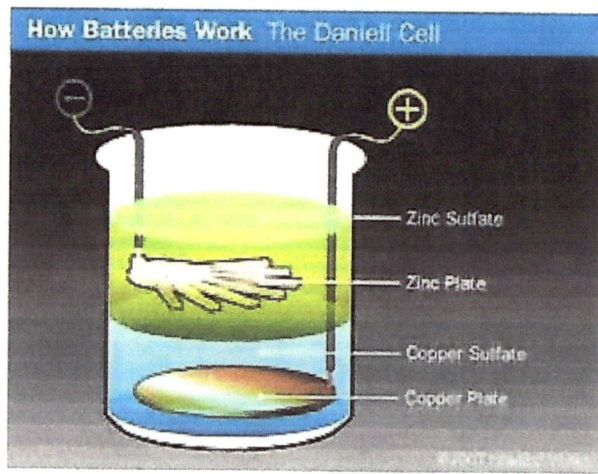

Crystal salt lamps bind excessive positive ions with their negative ions thus have positive therapeutic effects.

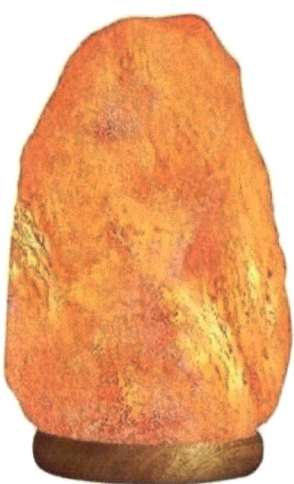

I have a Himalayan salt lamp that is beautiful. Every day when I turn it on I say, "Jesus, you are the light of the world." To me it's perfect because He is not only the Light of the World, He is the Great Physician. And He says that we are the salt of the earth. What more beautiful example of being salt than this salt lamp... warm, inviting, pure, healing, and healthy.

*These salt lamps are available through www.purehimalayansalt.com or
by calling (607) 281-4996 EST.*

Entire spas are built around the wonderful effects that Himalayan salt has on the body.

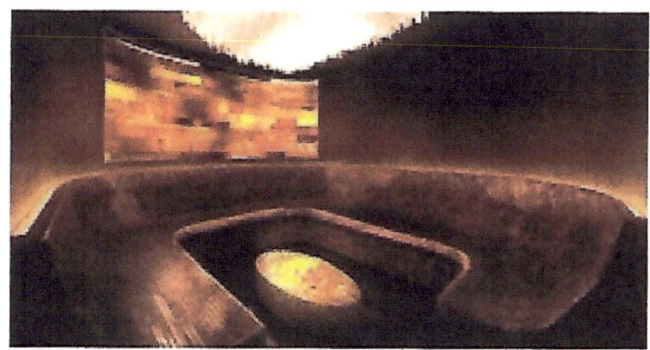

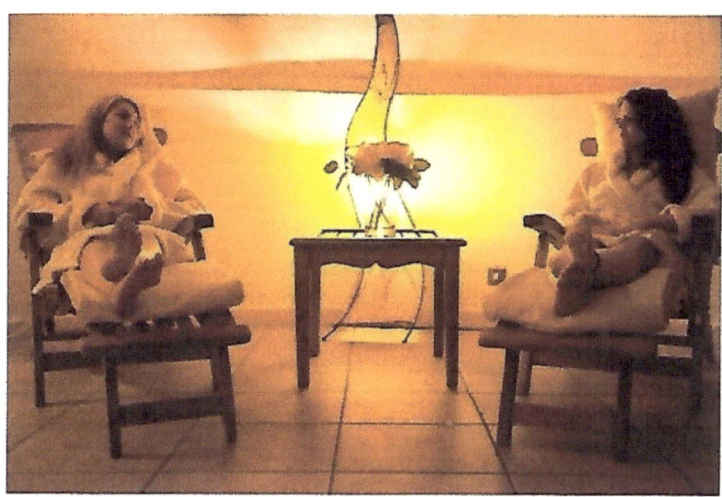

In summary, extraordinarily, salt's crystalline structure is electric, not molecular.

Due to its mutability, salt does not have to be metabolized by our body in order to be absorbed.

Osmosis, the foundation of cellular metabolism, is controlled by salt.

Without salt we could neither act nor think.

There is a wonderful book about Himalayan salt called <u>Water and Salt</u> by Dr. Barbara Hendel and Peter Ferreira. It reveals some of the intricacies and amazements of water and salt that I believe are worthy of our attention.

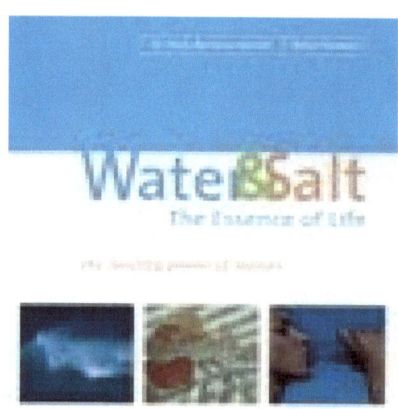

Available for purchase at either
www.purehimalayansalt.com
or at www.amazon.com

This is the quote by former President of the United States, John F. Kennedy, on the front jacket:

"All of us have in our veins the exact same percentage of salt in our blood that exists in the ocean, and, therefore, we have salt in or blood, in our sweat, in our tears. We are tied to the ocean. And when we go back to the sea...we are going back from whence we came."

I order my Himalayan salt by either calling (607) 281-4996 or by going their website at **www.purehimalayansalt.com.**

I am very pleased with the quality of their salt and their commitment to the profound importance of quality Himalayan salt in regard to our health. I usually get the five-pound bag of extra fine pink salt, which is $24.00.

The following pages are from Pure Himalayan Salt for your information regarding salt caves, spas and crystal salt tiles.

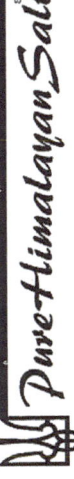
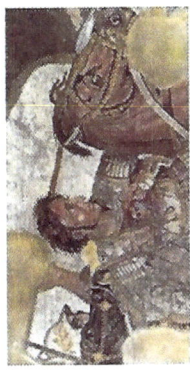

Pure Himalayan Salt

According to local beliefs, the Himalayan Salt Mines (also known as Khewra Salt Mines) were first discovered when Alexander the Greats' horses started kicking the ground covering the salt. Seeing that horses with flesh wounds were healing faster than expected, the soldiers began checking to see what the horses were unearthing. Thus the rich Himalayan Salt deposits were first discovered.

Pure Himalayan Salt crystals are comprised of the same colloidal minerals that are required by the human body in order to sustain life as described in the book Water and Salt the Essence of Life.

Today the Himalayan Salt Mines are the second largest Salt Mine in the world and are located in what is now the northern region of Pakistan.

Having crystallized over some 250 million years Pure Himalayan Salt was formed long before present day oil spills, chemical run-offs and toxins began flowing into our oceans.

Making Good Things Happen

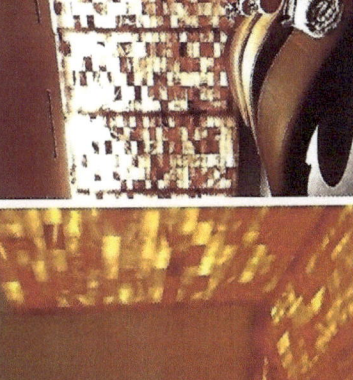
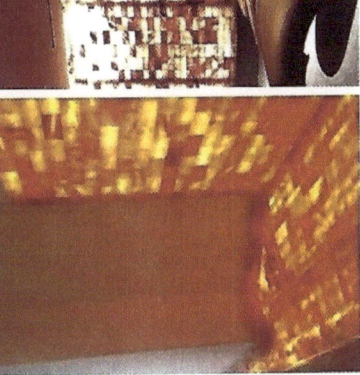

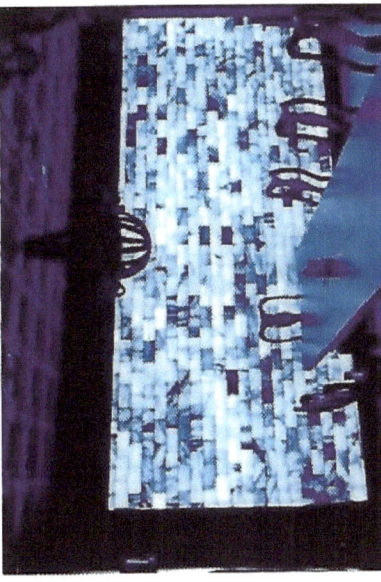

SALT CAVES
SALT SPAS
RESTAURANTS & BARS

TAKING A DREAM AND MAKING IT REAL

www.purehimalayansalt.com
(607) 281-4996
click4salt@gmail.com

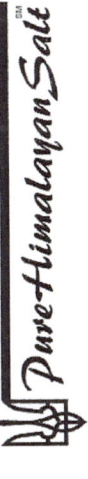

Pure Himalayan Salt

Being a gourmet cook and a Reiki Healer I started using Pure Himalayan Salt in cooking.. My love for Pure Himalayan Salt grew deeper as I started discovering the different ways I could use it and apply it to my daily life. What started as a "gourmet experience" turned into a way of life for me. Pure Himalayan Salt "feeds the body and fuels the soul."

Thinking about building a salt cave ?

at home? Or perhaps for the public? Email us your room dimensions and a design if one is available. Would you like salt tiles on the 4 walls? Or 3 walls or on two? On the ceiling? What would you like for flooring? Finished wood floor? Or perhaps salt tile? We are prepared to design, build and or supply the materials you will need to make your dream a reality. Pure Himalayan Salt, we make it happen for you.

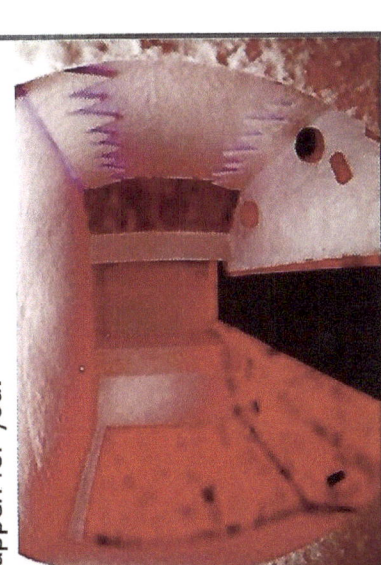

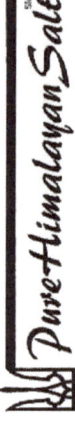

PureHimalayanSalt

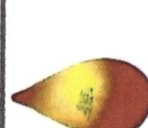
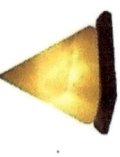
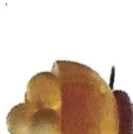

Like Us On
facebook f

Hand carved by skilled artisans the candleholders enhance the beauty of the home. As the candle is lit it gently heats the Himalayan Rock Salt illuminating the crystals and emitting negative ions into the air. Natural air fresheners and air purifiers the Himalayan Candle Holders highlight the home décor while casting an amber glow infusing the surroundings with positive energy and ambient glow.

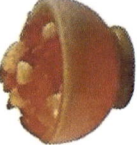
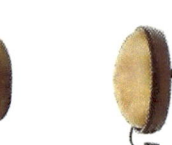
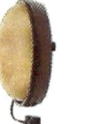
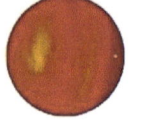
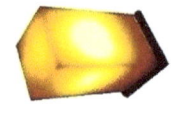
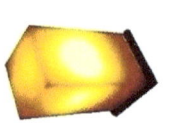

Each Pure Himalayan Salt Crystal Lamp is distinctly unique and one of a kind therefore no two pieces of Himalayan Crystal Salt are alike. Variations in color range from almost clear to light pink, orange then red and dark red. The same size and shape may register different weights. This is part of the living beauty of the Pure Himalayan Salt Crystal. Although the "same", each crystal has its own inherent personality, characteristics, look and feel.

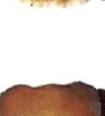
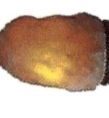
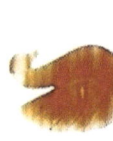
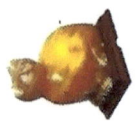

Himalayan Salt Lamps release negative ions into the air even when unlit. Once a heat source is applied, however the negative ionic output is increased (up to 600% as per Alpha Labs, Salt Lake City, Utah, USA). It is these negative ions that filter out free radicals, toxins, pollen and chemical impurities out of the air. Pure Himalayan Salt lamp naturally purifies the indoor air, creating an optimal air balance. Your Pure Himalayan Salt Lamp will not shrink or lose weight. To Clean: wipe with damp cotton towel. For Deep cleaning wipe with solution half water and half white vinegar. Allow to air dry.

www.purehimalayansalt.com
(607) 281-4996
click4salt@gmail.com

PureHimalayanSalt

Pure Himalayan Salt may be used in the kitchen, in the bath and throughout the home. Use this salt to make sole, for netti pots, sinus rinse and to refill salt pipes. Salt tiles are used to build salt caves, for cooking food and for foot detox.

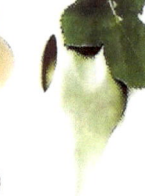
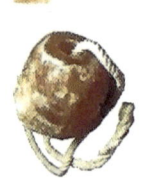
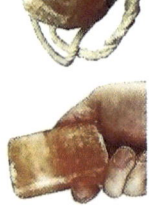
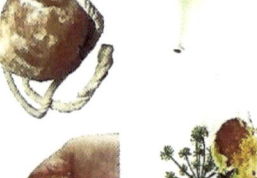
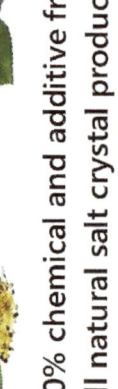

100% chemical and additive free. All natural salt crystal products

Salt therapy was prescribed by Hippocrates who recommended breathing in the steam from boiling water and salt. Today there are "salt spas" springing up in US cities—offering the healing environment of Himalayan Crystal Salt. When you bring Pure Himalayan Salt home whether in the form of a Tea Light Candleholder, Salt Lamp or Salt Rocks you are bringing home a piece of the ancient Himalayas.

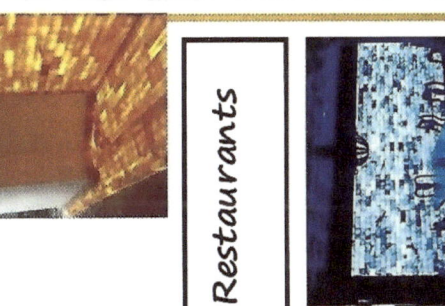
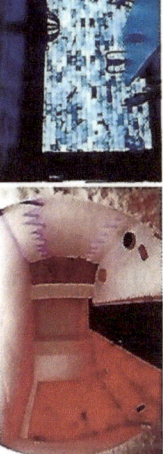
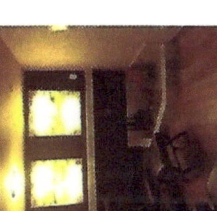
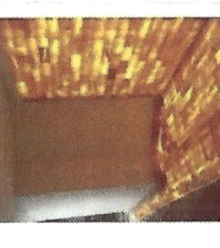
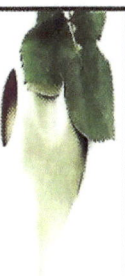
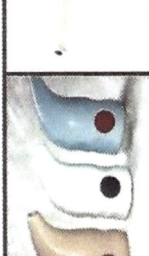

Panel 1 (right)

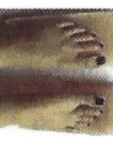

100% chemical and additive free

How To use the Himalayan Crystal Salt Foot Detox Tiles

- Place towel on floor.
- Heat oven to 250 degrees. Place tiles on cookie sheet or directly on oven rack and heat for approximately 20 minutes. Using oven mitts, remove tiles. The Pure Himalayan Salt slabs will be hot.
- Place hot tiles on prepared towel. Test the temperature of the salt tiles. If too hot lay another towel over the hot tiles and place feet on top.
- Due to the intrinsic properties of the Pure Himalayan Salt crystal bonds, the salt tiles will remain hot
- Relax, Unwind and Enjoy

Suggested Use: Great to use while sitting at the computer.

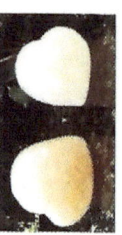
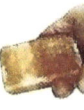

Click4salt@gmail.com
(607) 281-4996
www.purehimalayansalt.com

Panel 2 (middle)

Natures own
Massage salt rocks, Deodorants, Salt Soaps & Beauty Bars

Made from 100% Pure Himalayan Crystal Salt, *Pure Himalayan Salt* Bars and Salt Deodorants naturally contain 84 colloidal minerals described in the book "Water and Salt" and same as found in the human body. Chemical and additive free, they do not deposit aluminum on skin or any other man made chemicals. All natural, organic and pure.

Products so pure you can eat them.

Salt Beauty Bars & Deodorants

Apply to wet underarms by gently stroking one end of deodorant bar few times in armpit. When dry, the Pure Himalayan Salt Deodorant frms a natural barrier between human sweat and surrounding air thus in hibiting the growth of bacteria, and neutralizing unpleasant underarm odor.Shaped to easily fit into your hand, Pure Himalayan Salt Beauty Bars will last thru hundreds of uses (from 6 months to 2 years).

As a facial soap or for ionic bath soap:

Gently rub salt bar over wet face or use in shower or bath. Removing the outermost layer of dead skin cells Pure Himalayan Salt Bar leaves the skin revitalized, rejuvenated, replenished and radiating a natural glow.

Panel 3 (left)

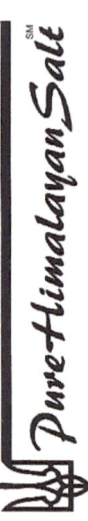

Pure Himalayan Salt is approved by the National Institute of Health and the FDA

No bleach

no anticaking agents

not sprayed with pesticides and toxins

Un-fumigated

Loading and unloading each sea container by hand we circumvent the required fumigation as applied to all palletized salt imports.

Salt therapy was originally prescribed by Hippocrates who recommended breathing in the steam from boiling water and salt. Today there are "Salt Spas" springing up all over US cities offering the healing therapeutic enviment of Himalayan Crystal Salt. Bringing Pure Himalayan Crystal Salt into your home one is remembering and reconnecting with the resonance of the ancient ocean that existed in the Himalayas millions of years ago.

Click4salt@gmail.com
(607) 281-4996
www.purehimalayansalt.com

STEP FOUR: PATHOGEN ELIMINATION

*This step helps build a good, healthy, fully functional **immune system.***

In Hulda Clark's book, <u>The Cure for All Diseases</u>, she states that

ALL DISEASE IS CAUSED BY POLLUTION OR PARASITES

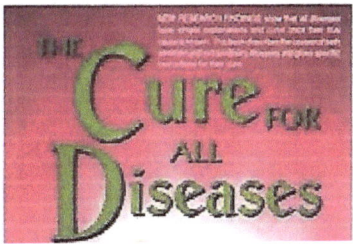
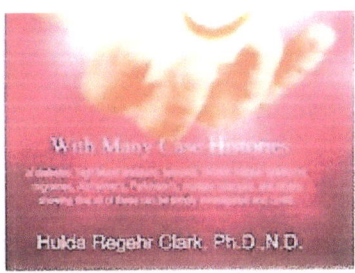

Pollutants are in the air, water, ground, and food we eat and cleaning products we use: mold, MSG, viruses, bacteria, artificial sweeteners and a host of other pathogens.

We ingest **parasites** on fresh produce, in undercooked fish and pork, through contact with cat feces, mosquito bites and by simply walking across the grass in bare feet.

These are all acidic and harm our bodies unmercifully.

This is how I learned about Immune 26:

In the middle of June 2002, every joint in my body ached. My energy level was pathetic. As I walked, I sighed. I didn't know what had happened to me but I knew if something didn't change, I wouldn't be able to go to my son's wedding at the end of the month.

I prayed. A friend I hadn't talked to for two years called and told me I had to talk to his uncle. His uncle was 59 at the time and a plumber by trade. He was taking cortisone shots in his shoulder because he couldn't lift his arm. His blood sugar level was over 300. In addition he was on three heart medications.

When he started taking what he called Immune 26 everything cleared up. And fast! In just three days! When I spoke with him he was doing karate with his grandchildren again.

I thought I'd give it a try. That was on a Wednesday. I ordered it that day. It arrived two days later on Friday. It came with a little tiny scoop. I didn't know how much to take but I knew it was egg powder. So I put one little scoop in soymilk, blended it up and took it Friday, Saturday and Sunday.

By Monday-three days later-- all the pain was out of my joints and I was able to go to my son's wedding and danced my feet off!

It also lessened the pain of fire ant bites on my feet substantially. The pain was gone in a couple of days instead of in a month. I continued to take it and shared it with great results.

After I realized what an astounding product it was, I took it to the diabetes support group at MUSC (Medical University of South Carolina).

The people there experienced a rapid and very significant improvement in their blood sugar levels.

I also shared Immune 26 with a friend who had suffered all his life with pain in his ankle because he broke his ankle three times, once when he was hit by a car as a young child. This is his story he wrote in March of 2013:

Well get your kicks with Immune 26. That's right. I got a great friend and her name is Christine Lauren. And she introduced me to the I26 powder and said it would get rid of the pain in my foot.

Well like everyone else I tried everything because I broke my ankle three times when I was a child. I was hit by a car and almost lost my left ankle. My mother begged the doctor to try to save the ankle over seventy years ago. I've been to doctors and they said surgery or a brace or amputate the foot. I have had pain over seventy years. When the doctors told me what they would do I didn't have much of a choice but to try I 26. I was drafted into the army at 21 but never got in because my ankle was so bad. I was strong as a bull too. But now thanks to I 26 I could kick a football with no problem. Thanks to I 26 if you don't know what to do with your money send it to me and I will buy some more I 26 so I can get my kicks.

Salvatore Ardito

So what is Immune 26?

Immune 26 is an innovative, hyper-immune egg product based on the concept of passive transfer of immunity and is supported by over 20 years and $50 million in research and development.

Immune 26 has been proven to help the human body fight chronic inflammation, the silent killer. It has also been proven effective in animals!

Inflammation
may be keeping you from feeling your best.

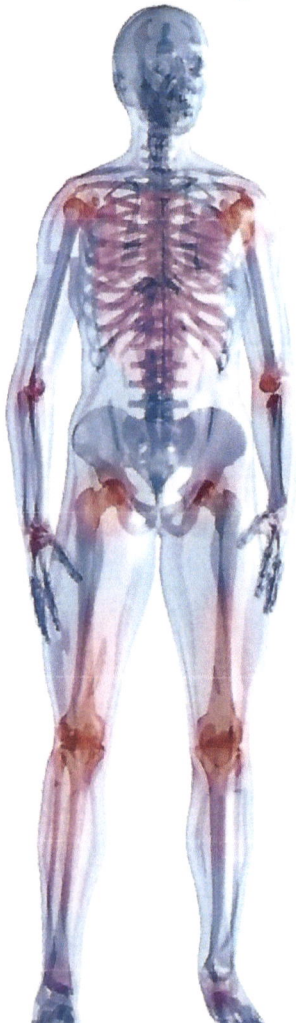

Are you sick and tired of feeling sick and tired? Doctors know that inflammation is at the root of most illness. In fact, 9 of the 10 deadliest diseases are caused by inflammation, and nearly everyone suffers from its day-to-day negative effects. Muscle and joint inflammation causes soreness and digestive tract inflammation causes cramps and bloating. More seriously, swelling of the arteries can cause heart health problems, while respiratory inflammation causes allergies and breathing difficulties.

i26 is the only supplement to help regulate inflammation by balancing the immune response. Inflammation is the tool the immune system uses to fight illness, but experts agree that too much inflammation is very bad for your health and too little can leave you unable to fight off illness and disease. All-natural i26 removes the guesswork and helps keep inflammation where it belongs.

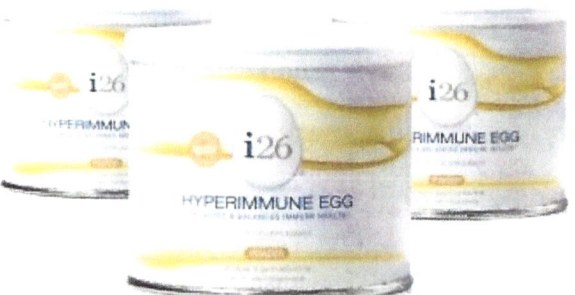

Complex immune factors delivered through 100% all-natural egg protein

i26 is the all-natural supplement that helps your body:

- Perform better
- Regulate the inflammatory immune response
- Reduce complications associated with inflammation

Don't just treat the symptoms. Help your body heal itself! While many products target the resulting symptoms of inflammation, i26 is the first of its kind to effectively balance improper immune inflammatory response. It has been proven to work in clinical and pre-clinical studies at Harvard and the U.S. Military, and in countless success stories every day.

Proven safe and effective:

- Over 100 patents and patent submissions worldwide
- Over 20 years and $50 million in research & development
- Listed in the Physicians' Desk Reference
- saGRAS File of Safety registered with the FDA

Help your body heal itself!

Youngevity   *   1-800-557-8477

We'll prove it to you. Try i26 for 90 days and see how your body will improve. If you're not completely satisfied, we'll refund your product cost. No questions asked. Remember, i26 is available exclusively from us.

ID#
101703963

You Love Your Pet...

and for as little as **20¢ A Day** you can give your pet the longest, healthiest and happiest life possible!

Companion FOR LIFE ® BY Legacy FOR LIFE

provides
Ultimate Nutrition
for your best friend...
with a taste they'll beg for!

Did you know Pet Ownership can help...

- lower blood pressure
- prevent heart disease
- lower human health care cost
- affect desire to succeed
- lower risk of eczema in babies
- better socialization
- reduce care giver stress
- provide mood therapy
- as therapy for stroke victims
- avoid loneliness
- increase self esteem
- sooth nerves
- psychological stability
- lower risk of allergies/asthma
- provide babies stronger immune activation
- reduce Alzheimer outbursts
- prompt more exercise
- provide safety and security
- heart attack patients live longer
- teach discipline
- reduce chances of child obesity by 50%
- reduce insurance premiums for the elderly
- fight depression
- as therapy for disabled

Let's face it! Pet ownership can improve your health!

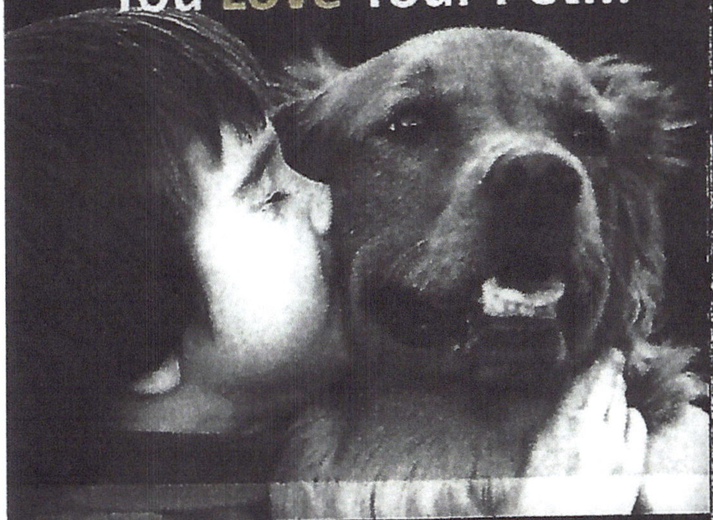

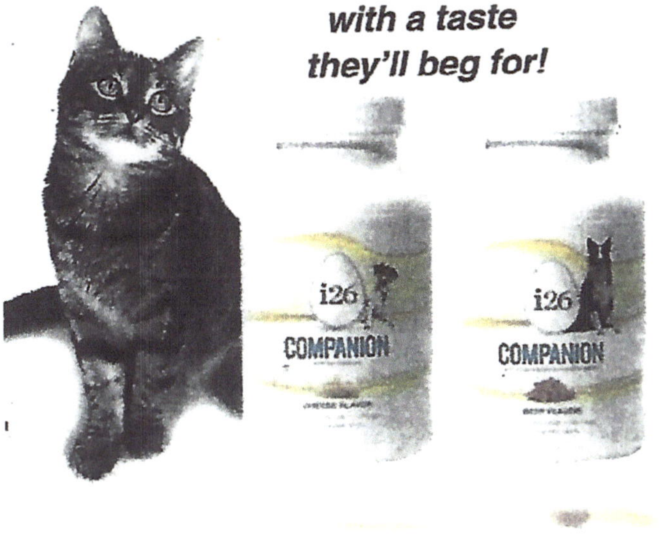

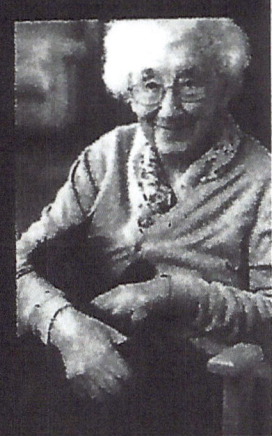

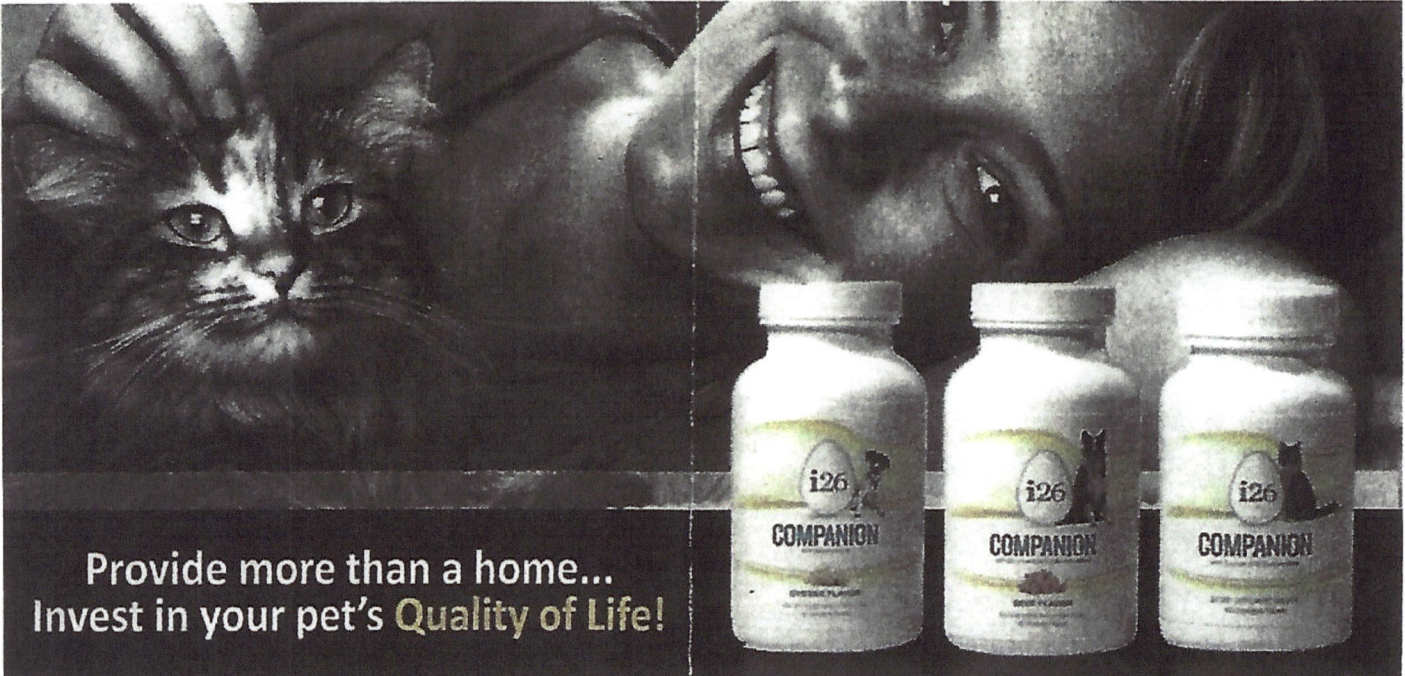

Provide more than a home...
Invest in your pet's Quality of Life!

Your pet will love getting them as much as you love giving them!

i26 Companion for Life® is a perfect whole food protein supplement, packed with essential vitamins and minerals. *Contains NO unnecessary fillers, corn, wheat, or soy. No animal by-products, hormones or harmful chemicals. Companion for Dogs® has added Glucosamine for healthy joints. Companion for Cats® has added Taurine to aid feline digestion.*

i26® is Pure Nutrition
"The Immune Solution" to meet all your family needs.

Protected by over 100 world-wide patents. Listed in the Physician's Desk Reference for Nonprescription Drugs and Dietary Supplements™ Backed by more than 2 decades and 50 million dollars in scientific research and development by two industry giants, ConAgra and Dupont

All intellectual property relating to Hyperimmune egg and i26 are now the property of Legacy For Life. The development team continues to produce Hyperimmune Egg and is part of Legacy for Life. Dupont and ConAgra visions are no longer directly associated with the product.

Buffet of Immune Components:

A balanced immune system protects health and wellness of the entire body. i26® supports and maintains a balance of:

*Cardiovascular Function
*Healthy Coat and Eyes
*Healthy Joints
*Digestion
*Circulatory System
*Peaceful rest
*Renewed Energy

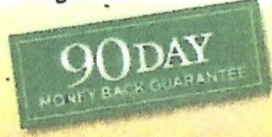

All Legacy products include a 90-day risk-free unconditional money back guarantee for new customers.

Most all creatures, great and small, love i26® and can feel and see results quickly.

Horses, cattle, sheep, exotic birds... even koi have found balance, health and wellness with i26® and Companion for Life®. *Note: For larger animals use pure i26® powder, or liquify for ingestion. Add one (1) scoop i26® per 300 lbs. of animal, and anticipate results!*

Cody's Story:

Sever Skin Disorder

"*The fur on my 10-year-old Siberian Husky, Cody, had been coming out due to a severe skin infection for about 16 months, leaving bare, irritated and pink skin on both sides of his body. We'd tried everything possible with the vets. Cody was lethargic, had lost a lot of weight, and we'd just about given up hope. Skeptical, we began giving Cody six COMPANION for Life Chewables per day. Within a month, Cody was feeling and looking much better; losing less fur. We began mixing i26® powder with yogurt (a treat he loves). Before long, Cody had regained weight, energy, and had a beautiful, healthy-looking coat.*"

Rosemary Baker

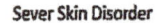
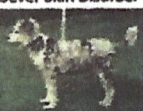

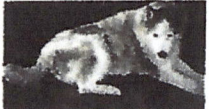

Skin Infection Virtually GONE!

A Picture of Perfect Health!

"*My fur-kids have been sooo healthy on i26® - my oldest has used it for 9 years! They all have beautiful coats, no skin disorders, bright eyes, and Samson (over 9 years old) still acts like a puppy full of energy! You would never know Lilah had an issue at one time where she virtually lost all her hair, due to an allergic reaction to fleas. ALL of it has come in beautifully, and, as you can see, her coat is flowing and healthy!*"

Livia Gail

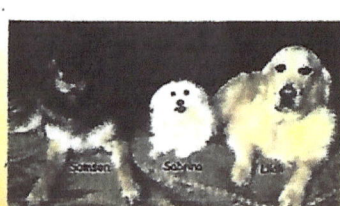

Here's what Vets using i26® to help their patients have to say:

"I have been highly impressed by the changes I have seen in so many of my patients. For example, recently an older dog with excessive weight was having difficulty getting around; he was lethargic and just slept all day. Knowing what i26 does for people, I added i26 Companion for dogs into its daily regimen.

Within less than a week, the dog was playing with the kids again and actively running up and down the stairs. I enjoyed the delight of the family and the children.

Because of their convenience, they and my other clients are thrilled to see i26 Companion Chewables on the shelves!"

Roger Baxter, DVM - Chinook, Montana
Large and Small Animal Practice
(f) President of the Montana
Veterinary Medical Association

"Support of immune function is important in maintaining health, and i26 appears to be unique in its ability to balance pro- and anti-inflammatory responses. As a practitioner that prefers using natural means to help primates, avians, and other exotics stay healthy, I find i26 has helped with my especially difficult cases."

Thomas I. Goldsmith DVM MS
Miami, Florida
Avian and Exotic Medicine

"I recommend i26 for the gastrointestinal health of calves and foals. Often by using i26 I have been able to help reverse decisions from owners to "put-down" animals. In terms of joint support, horses that were limping before demonstrate dramatic differences in their mobility and flexibility. Having i26 and i26 Companion available makes my day more productive, and a lot more enjoyable for my patients and family."

David L. Nirschi, DVM - Mohrsville, PA
Integrative Veterinary Practitioner
Bovine, Equine, Ruminants, and Exotics
Complimentary and Alternative Medicine

Pet Related Spending is Recession Proof

Spending on our pets has continued to climb for ten years with no end in sight. Pet owners happily cut other household and personal items from their budget to accommodate their beloved animal friends.

63% of American Households Have Pets

The average pet owner spends nearly $1500 per year on a dog; just over $1000 per year on a cat.

From organic foods and toys, doggie motels, spas and boutiques, to exclusive parks and events. Clothing, extravagant accessories; even steps to help pets access YOUR bed! People do not hesitate to spend money on pets they love. Americans are crazy about companion pets!

Pet owners spent in excess of 55 BILLION DOLLARS in 2011

Only YOU can share your pet's story. Help us share the gift of balance - i26® and Companion for Life® for dogs and cats.

Pets do not know placebos - their results cannot lie!

"In nearly two decades of marketing exceptional products, I've never had more fun... real fun, and made lasting friendships than when selling i26® to pets and their people. It's the easiest niche in marketing."
Pet People Are Happy People!
Connie Lewis, Oregon Coast

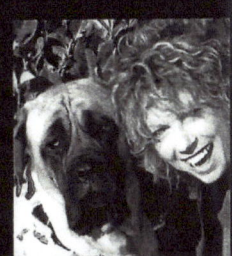

For more information about Legacy for Life products and opportunities to put you in biz with your pet(s), contact your Legacy Distributor:

Call Youngevity
1-800-557-5477
ID# 101703963

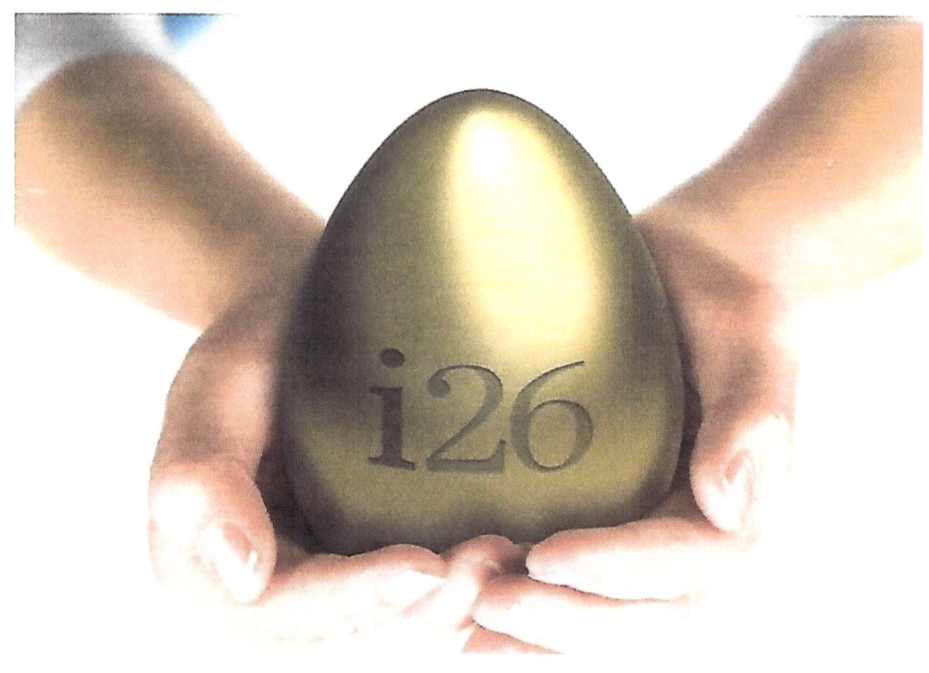

Immune 26 is one of the few health products that have been **double-blind placebo studied** and tested in clinics and universities all over the world.

Legacy for Life also has Immune 26 in shake form with vitamins called *Complete Support.*

To order Immune 26 call (800) 557-8477.

Developing i26, proving its efficacy, safety and benefits was no small proposition. i26 Hyper immune Egg was developed in the same manner that most pharmaceutical products are created.

More than $50,000,000 in research, development, pre-clinical and clinical trials, and patent costs was incurred. Also, there are over 100 patents and patent applications valued at over $35,000,000 protecting this technology. How many dietary supplements, or even pharmaceuticals, have even a fraction of these many patent instruments?

The claim that i26 supports the immune system by providing it with the "fuel" needed to function properly is supported by pre-clinical and clinical trials conducted on three continents. These pre-clinical and clinical trials have taken place at some of America's premiere institutions:

- o Harvard/Beth Israel Deaconess, Boston, MA
- o The Hospital for Special Surgery in NY, NY
- o The United States Military, Natick, MA
- o The University of Southern Mississippi, Hattiesburg, MS

The results of many of these studies have been published in leading scientific journals.

Testing results on the i26 Hyper Immune Egg have shown that it does:

Balance and support the immune system
Helps the body
* maintain cardiovascular function and a healthy circulatory system
* maintain digestive tract health
* modulate autoimmune responses
* maintain healthy and flexible joints
* support energy levels
* shorten exercise recovery times
* increase muscular strength, endurance, and stamina
* decrease heart rate during exertion
* reduce 2nd day soreness
* increase anaerobic peak power

Your immune system is involved in the health of every part of the body. When the immune system is functioning at an optimal level great health benefits are realized. Research is the basis for i26 and studies on specific benefits continue today.

How to Order

Ionizer Plus Water Electrolyzer

More information available at **www.hightechhealth.com**
High Tech Health is located in Boulder, Colorado.
Call (800) 794-5355 (toll free, Mountain Standard Time) to speak with any
High Tech Health Product Specialist to receive a substantial discount off
this wonderful product!
*Be sure to mention the name Christine Lauren or this book's title Health
Made Simple! for your discount.*

Barley Life

Contact **The A.I.M. Companies** in Nampa, Idaho at 800-456-2462 (MST). Just give
them my I.D. number as your sponsor, which is 39706. Best price for you if you sign
up as a member to purchase at wholesale. $100 in product waives the $20
membership fee. Herbal Fiberblend is also available through AIM. Additional
information at **www.barleylife.com**.

Himalayan Salt

You can order Himalayan salt by calling 607-281-4996 EST and ask for Natalie or by
going to their website at **www.purehimalayansalt.com**. I usually get the five-pound
bag of extra fine pink salt, which costs $24.

Immune 26

*Since this book was first begun, Legacy for Life has become a part of a larger company
called Youngevity. This has some very exciting advantages for you. Youngevity is an
umbrella company to a great variety of quality health and wellness products. So when
you order Immune 26 you can also get a discount on other great products. More below.*

To order Immune 26
Simply call **(800) 557-8477** to reach Youngevity (9am-6pm Monday – Friday PST). The
first time you call they will set up an account number for you as a **preferred customer**,
which gives you a **30% discount** off retail for all purchases. To be set up as a preferred
customer please give them my account number which is **101703963**.
This gives you the opportunity to shop the entire Youngevity website and get your
discount on every purchase. If you want to share this with others you can earn a
bonus on their purchases if you sign up as a **distributor**. This is a one-time $25
sign-up fee. No yearly renewal fees. No cancellation of your membership.

If you would like to share this great product with your friends and family or other amazing Youngevity products, click the "Join" button at the upper right corner of the screen. The first item is an "Enrollment Pak" for $25. This entitles you to bonuses if you give your distributor number to your friends and family and they make purchases under your name and number. This is the only time you will sign up. No yearly renewal fees. No cancellation of your account.

These bonuses apply to all the Youngevity products!
Over a thousand to date!

PLEASE NOTE: If you go to the LFLnewwave.youngevity.com site and another name appears as the Independent Distributor, be assured you are at the right website. This book was printed before the change was made to the author's name. Thank you.

Best wishes in attaining health made simple!

Christine Lauren

To order, search by author's name and title at
www.amazon.com and or use this web address
www.createspace.com/6112786 as an URL.
Do not put in the search bar.

Contact author at feetadancing@gmail.com

OTHER BOOKS AVAILABLE BY CHRISTINE LAUREN

Keys of the Kingdom Revealed
Have you ever wondered what the keys of the kingdom are and how to use them? This book will reveal the answers to you!   *To order go to www.createspace.com/6315809* as URL

Safety Inside the Circle- Save Sex for Marriage, But Why?
Bible based, but casually written as if in a conversation with the reader. Scripture references documented through footnotes. Includes an eighty-point questionnaire to determine if a relationship will work.
To order go to www.createspace.com/3498143 as URL

Seven Steps Out of Depression
Simply presented, yet effective in bringing hope through specific action steps. Bible based.
To order go to www.createspace.com/3644723 as URL

The ABCs of Jesus Coloring Book
An evangelism tool with scripture for each letter of the alphabet, teaching children who Jesus is plus a certificate to frame to celebrate the day of their salvation. Also includes a letter from Jesus welcoming them into His family. Available in four languages:
For English go to www.createspace.com/3514547 as URL
For French go to www.createspace.com/3577656 as URL
For German go to www.createspace.com/3633212 as URL
For Spanish go to www.createspace.com/3590244 as URL

The ABCs of Me Coloring Book
A wonderful evangelism tool with scripture for each letter of the alphabet that will teach children who they are in Christ. Also includes a certificate to frame to celebrate the day of their salvation and a letter from Jesus welcoming them into His family.
To order go to www.createspace.com/3643816 as URL

Stories & Poems of Faith, Wisdom and Kindness
This book is illustrated with color pictures and contains a wide variety of stories and poems for adults and children that will touch their heart and stir the spirit.
To order go to www.createspace.com/3549099 as URL

Wisdom Through Symbols
This book will challenge youth and adults to get their hands on Proverbs in a new way. Reader will work with scriptures as formulas for life expressed in symbols. One of the intents of this book is to show cause and effect regarding the happenings of life so that the reader will not be blindsided by what may come their way in this world.
To order go to www.createspace.com/3624757 as URL

TO ORDER go to www.amazon.com and put in the title of the book or use its web address as an URL.
Do not put in the search bar.
No minimum purchase required.
Books can be shipped in the United States & internationally.

Contact author at feetadancing@gmail.com